The *Social Communication Intervention Programme Resource* is accompanied by a number of printable online materials, designed to ensure this resource best supports your professional needs.

Go to https://resourcecentre.routledge.com/speechmark and click on the cover of this book.

Answer the question prompt using your copy of the book to gain access to the online content.

THE SOCIAL COMMUNICATION INTERVENTION PROGRAMME RESOURCE

The Social Communication Intervention Programme (SCIP) has been developed to support school-aged children (6–11 years) with social communication, pragmatic, and language needs. SCIP provides a rationale and method for providing specialist level pragmatics and language therapy for these children who have significant social communication differences.

The SCIP model is introduced in *The Social Communication Intervention Programme Manual*, and this book presents the content of the intervention programme itself, using a nested structure of 150 adaptable therapy activities. It contains the complete set of resources required to plan and deliver the interventions set out in the companion book, including forms, activities, and ready-made information sheets. Content can also be downloaded and printed for easy use.

Used alongside *The Social Communication Intervention Programme Manual*, this book offers a truly practical, tried-and-tested model to provide targeted, individualised intervention for children with social communication needs. It is an essential tool for speech and language therapists, specialist teachers, and psychologists who are working with children with social communication, pragmatic, and language needs.

For the most effective use, *The SCIP Resource* should be purchased alongside *The SCIP Manual*.

Catherine Adams is an Honorary Senior Lecturer in Speech and Language Therapy at the University of Manchester, UK. She has led a number of research projects on pragmatic and language needs in children as well as pioneering work on the effectiveness of social communication intervention.

Jacqueline Gaile is a Consultant Speech and Language Therapist in independent practice with over 30 years' experience of working with children with language and social communication needs. She was also Senior Research Speech and Language Therapist on the SCIP research projects at the University of Manchester, UK.

"It is rare to find such a comprehensive programme: the intervention plan is directly linked to child assessment with clear benchmarks for progression. It provides an integrated method for developing language structure, social understanding, and pragmatic skills."

Courtney Frazier Norbury, *Professor of Developmental Language & Communication Disorders at University College London*

"SCIP is the first evidence-based program to address the complex nature of social communication disabilities in children with autism, developmental language disorder, and social (pragmatic) communication disorder. The program provides detailed assessment and intervention activities for facilitating language processing, social, and pragmatic knowledge and skills. Guidelines and practical suggestions for the involvement of school staff and parents are included, so that children's new skills generalise to interactions with peers and family members. In short, SCIP is a must-have for professionals who want to comprehensively support children's social communication abilities."

Geralyn R. Timler, *Professor & Program Director, On-Campus Clinical SLP Program. Director, Social Communication and Language Evaluation (SCALE) Lab, James Madison University*

THE SOCIAL COMMUNICATION INTERVENTION PROGRAMME RESOURCE

SUPPORTING CHILDREN'S PRAGMATIC AND SOCIAL COMMUNICATION NEEDS, AGES 6–11

Catherine Adams and
Jacqueline Gaile

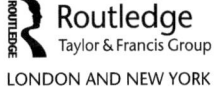

Routledge
Taylor & Francis Group

LONDON AND NEW YORK

Cover credit: Getty Images. Cover design: J Steer

First published 2024
by Routledge
4 Park Square, Milton Park, Abingdon, Oxon OX14 4RN

and by Routledge
605 Third Avenue, New York, NY 10158

Routledge is an imprint of the Taylor & Francis Group, an informa business

British Library Cataloguing-in-Publication Data
A catalogue record for this book is available from the British Library

ISBN: 978-1-032-70663-4 (hbk)
ISBN: 978-1-032-70660-3 (pbk)
ISBN: 978-1-032-70664-1 (ebk)

DOI: 10.4324/9781032706641

This book is also available for purchase as part of a set, ISBN: 9781032706672

Typeset in DIN Pro
by Deanta Global Publishing Services, Chennai, India

Access the Support Material: https://resourcecentre.routledge.com/speechmark

CONTENTS

PREFACE

Speech-language practitioners possess unique information about the 'how' and the 'what' of communication intervention but they rarely have the opportunity to write it down. As speech-language practitioners, we were aware of the need for a framework of intervention and a resource for children with complex and persistent social communication needs. In *The Social Communication Intervention Programme Manual and Resource* we present an evidence-based intervention for children with persistent social communication needs. In *The SCIP Manual* we provide a theoretical rationale and a method for integrated intervention with such children; in *The SCIP Resource* a large set of intervention activities from which individualised plans are created is presented in a nested structure reflecting SCIP's theoretical rationale. Procedures and content have been refined from the research version of *The Social Communication Intervention Programme Manual* and instructions for delivery of the phases of intervention have been developed more fully.

The purpose of engaging children, their parents, and school staff in SCIP Intervention is to enable children to be more confident communicators in the long term. The central goals of SCIP are to develop children's skills in pragmatics and language ability, grow their understanding of their own communication and interaction experiences, increase parents' and teachers' knowledge of the child's strengths and needs, and develop their ability to support the children when they face confusing or challenging communication experiences. Children are actively involved in evaluating communication and interaction experiences and generalisation of skills is built in from the start through personalised intervention planning.

Close working at all stages of SCIP is essential. Parents and teachers set goals jointly with the practitioner and where possible, the children themselves contribute to goal setting and considering progress. The intention of SCIP, therefore, is to develop opportunities with parents, teachers, and the children to enhance social communication experiences across middle and later childhood and beyond alongside building confidence and self-esteem.

There is now widespread recognition of the need to disseminate evidence-based intervention methods in the speech-language profession. Evidence-based methods that focus on pragmatics and social communication are relatively rare at present. SCIP Intervention is an approach to our practice that we wanted to share with other speech-language practitioners to the ultimate benefit, we hope, of the children and their families.

ACKNOWLEDGEMENTS

Many people were involved in the development of SCIP Intervention and the SCIP research studies. We acknowledge the contribution of Elaine Lockton, Catherine Aldred, Gillian Earl, and Jenny Gibson, who all helped shape our thinking about the organisation of intervention elements and contributed to the content of specific activities; Bonnie Brinton and Martin Fujiki provided essential encouragement for publication of the intervention; Jenny Freed, James Law, Kirsty McBean, and Marysia Nash for further support with the SCIP project. Thanks also to Catherine Bird, Sibyl Havens, Vivienne MacKenzie, and Rachel Stevens, whose energy and dedication allowed the evidence from the SCIP trial to be produced. Finally, we acknowledge with appreciation the children, schools, speech-language therapists, and families who were involved in the SCIP research studies and from whom we learned so much.

INTRODUCTION

The Social Communication Intervention Programme or SCIP is a communication intervention aimed at supporting children's needs in social communication, pragmatics, and high-level language processing. It is a specialist level intervention which is intended to be supervised by experienced speech-language practitioners. SCIP is aimed at children aged between 6 and 11 years of age.

The SCIP Resource contains

- ❖ over 150 speech and language intervention activities associated with the SCIP programme
- ❖ information sheets for parents/teachers
- ❖ bespoke resources for some activities
- ❖ suggested equipment lists
- ❖ SCIP Assessment to Intervention Map
- ❖ SCIP Intervention Planning and Record Form

The SCIP Resource should be used alongside ***The SCIP Manual*** which contains the background rationale, therapy methods, and instructions for the programme. **Using *The Resource* without knowledge of the method or individualised planning and therapy methods stated in *The Manual* will not be consistent with evidence-based practice.**

Summary of content in The SCIP Intervention Resource

The main purpose of *The Resource* is to provide the practitioner[1] with therapy activity content that can be used to support an individualised programme.

In order ***to plan intervention***, the practitioner will need access to *The SCIP Manual*.

Access to the SCIP Assessment to Information Map and to the SCIP Intervention Planning and Record Form (both in this *Resource*) will also be required. The process for planning intervention and selecting activities for the three Phases of SCIP Intervention is described in *The SCIP Manual*.

In order **to deliver intervention**, the practitioner will need to have read and understood the SCIP principles of intervention, therapy techniques, and specific metacognitive methods presented in *The SCIP Manual* and to select intervention activities from *The SCIP Resource*.

Intervention activities in this *Resource* should be used in conjunction with overall planning of intervention in Phases 1 and 2 as described in Chapters 8 and 9 of *The SCIP Manual*.

Organisation of The SCIP Resource
Phase 1 content and activities

The content of Phase 1 Intervention is shown first. Phase 1 activities are listed in the **Phase 1 Intervention content table**. This is followed by the Phase 1 activities shown in the order in which they appear in the content table.

The five **Phase 1 to Phase 2 pointer activities** are shown after the Phase 1 activities. Pointer activities are designed to assess how far the child's skill in this aspect of communication has progressed. At the end of Phase 1, the practitioner may decide to use a pointer activity in some or all of the Phase 1 Objectives. Pointer activities can provide further information, e.g., to determine how secure the core skills are, and indicate the need for further intervention in Phase 2 to consolidate these skills.

Phase 2 planning and the SCIP Assessment to Intervention Map

During Phase 1 and by the end of that phase, plans for Phase 2 individualised content are drawn up using the **SCIP Assessment to Intervention Map**. This is shown in three parts, corresponding to the main Components of Phase 2: Social Understanding and Social Interpretation (SUSI), Pragmatics (PRAG), and Language Processing (LP). The full version of the SCIP Assessment to Intervention Map is shown here and in *The SCIP Manual*. This contains guidance on assessment findings and reported information about each child and how to link these to specific Sections and Objectives within Phase 2 Intervention. A shortened version is also shown in this *Resource* as part of the Form.

Phase 2 activities

A **quick guide to Phase 2 activity targets** is provided on pages 55 to 66, to allow the practitioner to see the range of targets in each Component and Section during planning. These may also be useful for general record keeping of what has been delivered and achieved, for writing reports and for sharing with other professionals as needed.

A list of all Phase 2 Intervention content is shown in the **Phase 2 Intervention content table on pages 53 and 54.**

Phase 2 activities are then set out in the sequence: SUSI, PRAG, LP. For example, the complete content of the SUSI Component is shown first; then the content of SUSI 1 (Section) is shown; then all the intervention activities for SUSI 1 are set out in sequence as they appear in the Section Intervention content table. SUSI 1 is followed by SUSI 2, and so on.

In each Section (e.g., PRAG 2), intervention activities are preceded by an **Information Sheet.** This is a set of advisory instructions and tips written for parents and co-workers, to be used at the practitioner's discretion.

Therapy activities in The SCIP Resource

Activities in this *Resource* are numbered in a sequence which shows where each sits within the overall structure of the programme. Activities can be referred to just by numbers when familiarity with the content is reached, e.g., SUSI 2.1, Activity 2.

For example, each activity page starts with:

Phase and Component Name, e.g., Phase 2 SUSI
Section Number, e.g., SUSI 2
Objective Number and Objective Title, e.g., SUSI 2.1 Building emotion vocabulary

The activity number within that Objective and the activity title, e.g., Activity 2: Understanding vocabulary for intensity of feelings.

The activity content is then listed using a template of:

❖ purpose and target
❖ materials
❖ procedure

Some activities also contain instructions on how to simplify/extend the activity or how to personalise the activity.

Note that therapy activities in SCIP are described clearly to allow replication and supervised delegation. It is essential to understand therapy methods used in SCIP as well as how to combine therapy activities into an individual programme specific to the child's needs. For this, reading and applying the principles and procedures shown in *The SCIP Manual* are needed. Examples of how to select activities within a child's programme are shown in Chapters 8 and 9 and in the case study in *The SCIP Manual*.

The SCIP Intervention Planning and Record Form

The complete Form is shown at the end of this *Resource*. Contents of the Form are referred to in the planning chapters in *The SCIP Manual*. Examples of how to use the Form are shown in *The Manual* chapter on assessment and in the planning chapters (8–10).

Equipment and materials used in SCIP Intervention

Each activity lists the materials needed. In most cases, these materials are widely available published resources and examples of equipment and materials used in the SCIP trial are listed in Table 11.1. For some Objectives, the SCIP trial team created novel and bespoke resources to fit the requirements of particular activities. These are listed as Activity Resources and are presented in sequence with the activity.

Note that most activities require plain paper or white card, pens of various colours, and sticky notes in addition to specified materials. Hand puppets were used widely in the SCIP trial to act as partners in the intervention activities. A selection of puppets that can demonstrate different skills and needs is recommended, e.g., rabbit can be a good listener shown by his big ears, or a poor listener because he hops around thinking about other things.

Reference is made to 'workbooks' in many activities. These are simple notebooks in which materials and worked examples can be kept together. The practitioner can create different workbooks for parts of the intervention or one single workbook.

Examples of the workbooks that may be required are:

'Friendship book'
'Book of Feelings'
pragmatics 'rules' workbook
vocabulary workbook

Recommended general materials to support SCIP Intervention delivery

Home-School Book (can be a simple notebook)
Notebooks to record the child's work
Blank white paper
Blank white cards (index size, approximately)
Pens in red, blue, green, and black ink, colouring pens, and highlighting pens
Child-friendly glue
Sticky notes in standard square, speech bubble, thinking bubble, arrow, and star shapes, and different colours
A variety of 'reward' stickers and stamps (self-inked), e.g., 'keep going', 'well-done'
A selection of hand puppets (animals, people)

A selection of characters: boy, girl, animals, people in the child's life, presented as either small toys or as laminated cut-out pictures

Sheet of paper with speech bubbles in two columns

Examples of games and other resources

Snail's Pace Race (Ravensburger)

Manic Martians (Early Learning Centre)

Fuzzy Felt (various) (John Adams)

Character pictures of TV and cartoon characters, and magical creatures

Traditional stories and fairy tales (pictures to use as sequences)

Published speech and language therapy resources used in the SCIP Intervention

Resource (author)	Available from
Winslow Resources Colorcards: Skills for Daily Living: Social Behaviour cards Colorlibrary vocabulary sets Colorcards: Verbs Tell Me About It sequence set Verbal Reasoning Activities (DeGaetano)	http://www.winslowresources.com/
Black Sheep Press Talkabout Friends Talkabout School Picture Sequences (3–8 items) Practical Pragmatics Speech bubbles	http://www.blacksheeppress.com
Schubi picture sequences Sentimage Combimage	https://www.westermann.de/artikel/ L12036/SENTIMAGE-Bilderboxhttps:// www.westermann.de/suche?o=relevanz &q=Combimage
Fun Decks Emotions Multiple meanings Why – Because	http://www.superduperinc.com
Think It Say It – Improving Reasoning and Organisation Skills (Luanne Martin)	http://www.proedinc.com
120 Idioms at Your Fingertips (June Nicols and Susan Armstrong)	Various sources
What did you say? What do you mean? (J. Welton & J. Telford)	Various sources
Introducing Inference (Marilyn Toomey)	Various sources
Reading Comprehension Key Stage 1 Stories	http://www.schofieldandsims.co.uk
Scholastic Comprehension Practice workbooks (ages 5–10 years)	http://shop.scholastic.co.uk/products
Mixed Up Fairy Tales (Hilary Robinson & Nick Sharratt)	Available from bookstores
You Choose (N. Sharratt & P. Goodhart)	
Room on the Broom (Julia Donaldson)	
Playmobile sets	Various sources
Guess Who Game	Various sources
GLS: Learning To Sequence 4 Scene Sets	https://www.glsed.co.uk/product/curricular/ english/speaking-and-listening/learning- to-sequence-4-scene-sets-pack-of-48/ g1004115

Note

1   For brevity, the words he/his/him will be used to reference the child; the words she/her will be used to reference the practitioner.

PHASE 1 RESOURCE

The Phase 1 Intervention content table provides an ***overview*** of the content of Phase 1 in its entirety.

The Table shows the five Phase 1 Sections arranged in columns and their short codes (CM, USC) which are used to identify intervention activities quickly. Boxes in the Phase 1 Intervention content table show the Objectives for each Section. In Phase 1 each Objective has one intervention activity.

Phase 1 Intervention activities can be found in the following pages, in the order they appear in the Intervention Content Table (one Section at a time). Each activity states its required materials, purpose, and target. For Phase 1 Objective USC, SCIP Resources are presented in sequence with the activity. An Information sheet for Phase 1 is provided to share with parents and teachers, as required.

Phase 1 Intervention Content Table

Phase 1 Section	Phase 1 Objectives/activities
Comprehension monitoring (CM)	CM 1: Understanding the concept of knowing and not knowing CM 2: Understanding the concepts of guessing and working out CM 3: Strategies to signal non-comprehension CM 4: Asking for repetition
Introduction to understanding social context (USC)	USC 1: Making simple inferences from familiar sequences plus Resource USC 2: Identifying social context from behaviours and language plus Resource USC 3: Describing behaviours and language for social contexts USC 4: Simple personal reflection
Basic metapragmatic awareness (MPA)	MPA 1: Listening for content MPA 2: Understanding behaviours associated with listening MPA 3: Developing metapragmatic vocabulary MPA 4: Listener-speaker role-play
Basic narrative (BN)	BN 1: Understanding vocabulary for sequencing BN 2: Making simple inferences from pictures BN 3: Simple sequencing BN 4: Simple personal stories
Introduction to emotions in context (EM)	EM 1: Matching pictures and symbols to facial expressions EM 2: Linking emotions to events EM 3: Emotions ladder EM 4: Making inferences from facial expression and eye gaze

DOI: 10.4324/9781032706641-2

SCIP Phase 1

Phase 1 Information

The purpose of Phase 1 activities is to establish baseline core skills that are required for future intervention and to provide detail on your child's skills so as to assist with more accurate individualised planning for Phase 2 Intervention.

Phase 1 includes Objectives in

❖ Comprehension Monitoring (CM)
❖ Introduction to Understanding Social Context (USC)
❖ Basic Metapragmatic Awareness (MPA)
❖ Basic Narrative (BN)
❖ Introduction to Emotions in Context (EM)

Comprehension monitoring teaches your child to recognise when he has not understood a spoken instruction and to use a simple phrase to ask for repetition or clarification. Strategies to reduce guessing are practised and encouraged. **Understanding social context** teaches how spoken language and behaviour relate to the context/situation. In **Basic metapragmatic awareness** your child will learn the concept of active listening and will be taught key phrases to help him/her monitor whether he/she is using active listening skills or not. **Basic narrative** develops your child's ability to sequence and tell a story of three simple steps and builds towards being able to report simple events that he/she has recently experienced. He/she will be supported to understand and tell details related to 'who was there', 'what happened', and 'where the events took place'. **Introduction to emotions in context** ensures your child knows words, symbols, and facial expressions for the emotions happy, sad, angry, and scared. A simple visual representation of emotions using a ladder to represent that feelings change from OK at the bottom of the ladder to either happy, sad, angry, or scared will be used.

Throughout Phase 1, the practitioner will observe your child and gather information on your child's strengths and needs and use these observations to fine-tune the planning for Phase 2 Intervention if necessary.

How you can help

Work in Phase 1 of SCIP Intervention adds to the information available for Phase 2 planning as well as building core skills that will be needed for Phase 2 Intervention. Regular liaison with your practitioner, e.g., through the Home-School Book, will enable you to learn about new skills and strategies your child is being taught and to share information with your practitioner on how your child is responding to the teaching. Some additional practice will be required, and you will be invited to engage in using games, strategies, and key phrases at home and in school to assist your child in generalising new skills to everyday settings.

SCIP Phase 1

CM 1

Comprehension monitoring

Activity 1: Understanding the concept of knowing and not knowing

Purpose and target

To help the child understand the concepts of knowing and not knowing and practise ways to signal confusion or misunderstandings and ask for help.

Materials

Opaque box or tin with a lid.

Variety of familiar objects in a separate bag small enough to fit in the box.

Symbols for 'I know' and 'I don't know' for each person/puppet.

Paper and pens to create chart of helpful strategies.

Puppets to act as participants who take turns with the child.

Procedure

Explain the purpose is to learn words to help us talk about knowing and not knowing.

Hidden from view but with the child's knowledge, hide an object in the box.

Ask, "Who **knows** what's in the box?".

State, "I know" and explain how you know, i.e., "I put it there".

Give an 'I don't know' symbol to the child and the puppets.

Give yourself an 'I know' symbol and explain why.

Discuss ways of *working out* what's in the box – take a look/ask a friend/use a clue (semantic).

Each participant has a turn to work it out using one of the offered options.

When each participant knows, swap his card and explain explicitly what is happening, e.g., "Jack *knows* because *he had a look*".

Discuss at the end of every turn who knows and who still needs to work it out, swapping cards as participants know.

On one turn demonstrate that the puppet knows because he was listening to the child and explain that we can find out by listening to friends.

Provide praise for saying, "I don't know", e.g., "That's the right answer, you don't know – would you like to work it out?".

Continue around the group until each participant has an 'I know' symbol and describe all the ways used to work it out.

This activity depends on positive encouragement to say, "I don't know" and on demonstrating that it is possible to work things out in a variety of ways.

Discourage guessing, but if the child persists in guessing, move to CM Activity 2.

Role-reversal

After sufficient modelling, ask the child to hide the object and give out the symbols.

SCIP Phase 1

CM 2

Comprehension monitoring

Activity 2: Understanding the concepts of guessing and working it out

Purpose and target

To help the child understand the difference between guessing and working out, and replace unhelpful guessing with asking for help.

Materials

As for CM Activity 1 but use new objects.

Procedure

As for CM Activity 1.

Explain the purpose to the child as learning words related to 'guessing' and 'working out'.

Say that you are going to 'have a go' by 'guessing' what is in the box and not using a clue.

Ask the puppet to hide something in the box as before, out of view.

On a sheet of paper draw 2 columns, one for you and one for the child.

Give yourself ten guesses and get it wrong each time, marking each guess using an 'x' or a sad face.

Ask the child to 'work it out' by asking for a clue; he should be able to work it out in less than ten clues, but if not, help the child as needed to work it out.

Talk about the amount of 'work' each person had to do and show this visually using the list.

Compare the sad faces or 'x' marks for your guesses and the smiles for his working out.

Discuss the feelings that accompany getting it wrong by guessing, and draw sad or frustrated faces to match feelings alongside the wrong answers.

Role-reversal meta-challenge

Repeat asking the child to guess and offer as many guesses as they would like.

Ensure the child does not see the object being hidden and that it is not easy to guess.

Discuss how the child is feeling about guessing.

Ask the child if they wish to continue with guessing or try the strategies practised and continue.

If any child gets it right by guessing, explain that sometimes it is worth having a go – you might be lucky – but reinforce that the amount of work needed to guess is usually more than working it out.

If children do not want to guess, discuss why it is not always helpful and discuss what they could do instead.

This activity depends on repeatedly naming the behaviours of *thinking about the clues*, *working out* and *guessing*, and explaining and modelling the effects of each.

SCIP Phase 1

CM 3

Comprehension monitoring

Activity 3: Strategies to signal non-comprehension

Purpose and target

To help the child create visual reminders of strategies learned to signal non-comprehension and ask for clarification.

Materials

One large sheet of white card.
Coloured pens.

Procedure

Divide the sheet of card into two columns.

Draw a green traffic light on the left and write "I know" as the heading and in the column write/draw "keep listening", "keep working".

In the right column, draw a red traffic light and write "I don't know".

Add symbols or drawings to represent each idea.

Revise and discuss strategies to signal non-comprehension covered in CM1 and CM2 and add them to the "I don't know" column.

Remind the child of helpful words and phrases to use when he doesn't understand, e.g., say "I'm stuck" or "I don't know", or "Can you help me?", "I need a clue", etc.

If the child needs to be reminded not to guess, add a symbol for guessing and one for working it out, which will be preferred.

Allow the child to add his own words/drawings and examples.

Check the child's ISCP for examples of ways the child currently reacts when he doesn't understand and incorporate relevant actions/vocabulary into this activity.

SCIP Phase 1

CM 4

Comprehension monitoring

Activity 4: Asking for repetition

Purpose and target

To allow the child to practise asking for repetition; to support development of understanding that there are different reasons for not understanding an instruction.

Materials

Puppet.

Playmobil play scene or small life-like characters and scene.

Child's chart of comprehension monitoring strategies created in CM3.

Procedure

Use the puppet to give instructions to the child.

Explain that the puppet is going to ask the child to set up the Playmobil scene so that they can play together.

Operate the puppet to give a few simple instructions to start and the child can follow easily.

Puppet then deliberately changes some of the instructions in one of the following ways:

> coughs over a key word
>
> speaks too quietly
>
> uses nonsense words
>
> turns away and speaks to the wall or floor
>
> speaks too quickly

Observe the child's reactions and assist him to say, e.g., "I don't know what you mean", and to ask for repetition,

If child attempts to carry out incomplete instructions, make the meta-challenge explicit by saying, "You probably didn't hear puppet properly because he coughed. Would you like him to tell you again?". Model a phrase for the child to use if needed.

If the child persists in guessing, direct him to his chart to select an alternative, facilitatory strategy.

Observe how the child reacts to not understanding an instruction and add this to his ISCP. Inform parents and staff to note these responses as indications of times when the child is confused and how to assist with helpful strategies.

SCIP Phase 1

USC 1

Introduction to understanding social context

Activity 1: Making simple inferences from familiar sequences

Purpose and target

To help the child make simple inferences and describe actions and interactions in familiar social sequence pictures.

Materials

Schubi Tell Me About It Sequence sets 13 (swimming pool), 16 (getting ready for school), 17 (bedtime), or similar

USC1 Resource of scripts for social interactions in sequence sets.

Or three equivalent sets of pictures of familiar events in sequence with related narrative.

Procedure

Explain the task – "We are looking for clues in pictures to work out what might be happening".

From each of the three sequence sets, select one picture that gives the most obvious clue to the activity and lay these three pictures on the table. Ask the child to select the picture showing the children going to bed.

Discuss all relevant clues in the picture, e.g., "Here the children are in bed and Mum is reading a story. This usually happens before the children fall asleep".

Turn this card over and ask the child to find the children going swimming and discuss as before.

Repeat with the third picture (school).

Repeat twice more with three different pictures from each set. Each time select a picture which gives less obvious information than the first set.

Discuss all relevant clues in detail as before so that the child has a good overview of the inferences made, interactions between characters, and actions taken by each.

Now take one complete sequence, e.g., going swimming, and lay it out in order explaining as you lay it out, "Now we are going to work out what these people are saying and doing".

Describe the pictures one at a time, including for each picture a comment on who is in the picture, where they are and how you know (inference), and what is happening.

Use the prepared scripts in the USC1 Resource to add spoken language for the characters.

Invite the child to join you in providing a description of words and actions after you have started, and he knows what to do.

Model the phrase, "I think s/he's saying XX", giving reasons alongside and pointing out clues to inferences as needed.

Tell the story together until the end of the sequence pausing to allow the child to show what they know and what they can predict from the scenes.

At the end, ask questions, such as, "Who do you think might be saying XX?".

Repeat with the other sequences, asking the child to tell the story with/without support.

Gradually ask more difficult questions, e.g., to make predictions, work out what happened before a scene, and giving reasons for these predictions.

SCIP Phase 1

USC 1 Resource

Introduction to understanding social context

Activity 1 Resource: Making simple inferences from familiar sequences

Scripts for social interactions in sequences

Read the following scripts to the child making sure to denote any changes in speaker.

Set 16 Getting ready for school script

Picture 1 – Waking up.

The alarm clock is ringing to wake up the children so they can get ready for school. The children are sleepy. Harry says, "I'll switch off the alarm clock". Alice yawns and stretches.

Picture 2 – Washing.

The children are having a wash. "Please can you pass me a towel?" says Alice. "No problem, here it is", says Harry.

Alice dries her face then the children go to their room to get dressed.

Picture 3 – Getting dressed.

The children are putting on their clothes. "Have you seen my blue socks?" Alice shouts to her mum. Alice finds her socks in the drawers. "Hurry up!" says Harry, "I'm getting hungry".

Picture 4 – Eating breakfast.

Harry is happily eating his toast. "Be careful while I'm pouring the tea!" says Mum. Dad is just leaving for work. "Have a nice day everybody", he says.

Picture 5 – Cleaning teeth.

Harry and Alice are cleaning their teeth after breakfast. "Be quick!" says Alice. "We don't want to miss the bus!". They rinse out their mouths and run downstairs.

Picture 6 – Leaving the house.

Mum is waving goodbye to the children. "Have you got all your books?" she asks. "Don't worry Mum", says Alice. "We checked our bags last night". "Have a good day", says Mum. "Bye", say Harry and Alice. "Bye", says Mum.

Set 17 Getting ready for bed script

Picture 1 – Suppertime.

Mum, Dad, and the children are eating supper. Mum says, "Who wants some more bread?". "Me please", says Kim. "I'd like some more bread too", says Dad. "I want to make a jam sandwich".

"I'm going to have cheese on mine", says Kim.

Picture 2 – Putting on pyjamas.

It's time for the children to get undressed and put on their pyjamas. They race to see who can get ready first. "I've won!" shouts Kim. "Mum says we should put our dirty clothes into the laundry basket", says Ben.

Picture 3 – Having a wash.

The children are having a wash and cleaning their teeth before bed. Ben is having fun with the soap. "Look at all these bubbles!" he says. "Don't splash me!" says Kim.

Picture 4 – Choosing the story.

Kim and Ben are curled up in their beds. They are cosy and warm. "Which story would you like tonight?" says Mum. "The dragon story is my favourite", says Kim.

"I like that one too", says Ben.

Picture 5 – Listening to the story.

The children are listening to their bedtime story. "Can we have another one?" asks Ben when Mum has finished. Mum says, "No more stories. It's a school night".

Mum kisses them goodnight. "Goodnight", says Kim. "Sleep tight!" says Ben.

Picture 6 – Fast asleep.

The children are in bed. Mum has turned off the light and has gone downstairs.

Ben is snoring. Kim is cuddling her teddy bear.

Set 13 Going swimming script

Picture 1 – Packing for the day at the pool.

Here we have Mum and the children, Jacob and Anne, getting ready to go swimming.

The children are excited and are helping Mum to pack a picnic and their swimming gear. Mum says, "Jacob, have you got your swimming trunks?". Jacob says, "Yes Mum, here they are".

Picture 2 – Setting off on the bikes.

The children want to ride their bikes to the swimming pool, so Mum says, "OK, let's get our helmets on". The children get their helmets and get on their bikes. They wait until everyone is ready. Mum says, "Stay behind me and remember to stop at the red light".

Picture 3 – Arriving at the pool.

The children have arrived at the pool, and they need to buy their tickets. Mum goes to the counter and says, "One adult and two children for the pool, please". Mum pays the woman and collects the tickets and some change for the lockers.

Picture 4 – Getting changed.

Mum and the children go into the changing rooms. Mum asks another woman nearby, "How much is it for the lockers?" She puts all the clothes and shoes into the locker and finds a coin in her purse. "Come on", says Anne, "I'm getting cold".

Picture 5 – Swimming.

"Look at me, look at me!" says Jacob, "I can swim!" Anne loves her rubber ring. Mum says, "Don't go too deep". Jacob is splashing and laughing. He has found a new friend to play with.

Picture 6 – Ice cream.

After swimming for a while, the children ask Mum for an ice cream. "What flavour do you want?" asks Mum. "Vanilla for me", says Anne. "I want chocolate", says Jacob. "Oh no! I dropped mine, it's not fair!" says Anne. "I want another!"

SCIP Phase 1

USC 2

Introduction to understanding social context

Activity 2: Identifying social context from behaviours and language

Purpose and target

To support the child in understanding and recognising behaviours and language used in specific social contexts.

Materials

Pictures of different social contexts, e.g., swimming pool, library, birthday party, classroom, café, supermarket, hairdresser's, shoe shop, assembly, playground.

USC 2 Resource of scripts to describe social contexts by expected behaviours or language used in these situations.

Procedure

Explain the activity as one in which we "work out where something might happen".

Lay out a selection of the cards.

Describe the classroom by expected behaviours, e.g., the children are sitting on their chairs, the teacher is speaking to them. Ask the child to find the one you described.

Discuss reasons why it is the classroom – i.e., that this is what often happens in class.

Describe another context using the scripts in USC 2 Resource.

Ask the child "Where am I?". The child wins cards as he works out the context from the described behaviour.

Repeat using the same cards and explain that we are now thinking about "what people might say".

Give a simple example of what someone might say to start the new round.

Repeat until the child has won all cards using simple or more complex examples as required.

Add abstract and unfamiliar contexts as needed.

SCIP Phase 1

USC 2 Resource

Introduction to understanding social context

Activity 2 Resource: Identifying social context from behaviours and language

Scripts for social situations

Expected behaviours and spoken language are listed for each scene and include simple and obvious phrases, as well as some that require some inference and knowledge about the events.

Swimming pool

Behaviour	Language
I'm taking my clothes off and putting them in my bag	I can't open my locker
I'm putting my swimming trunks on now	Where do you put your clothes?
All my clothes are in the locker	How much do you need for the locker?
I'm splashing my sister	I forgot my towel
	I don't need armbands anymore

Birthday party

Behaviour	Language
Everyone is running around some chairs waiting for the music to stop	Let's sing Happy Birthday
	Can I open my present now?
We are sitting on the carpet passing a parcel around	It's time for the cake
Everyone is singing 'Happy Birthday'	I didn't get a chair this time, I'm out
Someone is blowing out the candles	I hope we play pass the parcel
	I don't like jelly

Library

Behaviour	Language
Everyone is sitting quietly reading a book	Can I borrow this book please?
Some people are searching the Internet	This book is four days late
A man is reading the newspaper	Quiet, no talking please
A little boy is playing with a train with his mummy	Everyone needs a ticket to borrow a book

Classroom

Behaviour	Language
Children are sitting at their tables	Excuse me, Miss, I'm finished
Some children are writing, and some are drawing	May I choose now?
A boy has put his hand up	Sienna took my pencil
A girl is collecting whiteboards	Tomas, can you give out the pens please?
	What lesson is after lunch?

Café

Behaviour	Language
People are sitting at tables eating and drinking	The menus are on the tables
A man is choosing a drink from a list	Did you order some tea?
A woman is asking for a clean fork	I would like the chocolate cake
People are reading the menu	Please may I have the bill?

Hairdresser's

Behaviour	Language
A girl is having her hair washed	How much is a trim?
People are sitting in front of large mirrors	This is the latest style
A woman has curlers in her hair	Would you like hairspray?
A man is having his hair trimmed	Would you like it a bit shorter?

Shoe shop

Behaviour	Language
A boy is walking around the shop in a new pair of trainers	Are these shoes comfortable?
	I'm going to measure your feet
A girl is looking at her shoes in a mirror	Do you need shoes for school or sport?
A woman is measuring a little boy's feet	Can I help you?
People are looking at the shelves	What size do you take?

Assembly

Behaviour	Language
Children are sitting in rows	Good morning children
A teacher is talking	Quiet please, everyone
A girl gives out song books	I have certificates for Year 2 children who completed the story-writing challenge
Everybody sings a song	

Playground

Behaviour	Language
Children are shouting and laughing	Can I play?
Some children are playing football	Pass me the ball!
Some children are swapping stickers	It's time for the bell to go
A helper is talking to a boy who has fallen	Where is the teacher?
Two girls are chatting in a corner	Can we play for a bit longer?

SCIP Phase 1

USC 3

Introduction to understanding social context

Activity 3: Describing behaviours and language for social contexts

Purpose and target

To help the child describe social contexts by expected behaviours and language, including social contexts that he finds challenging.

Materials

Pictures of social contexts and scripts, as for USC Activity 2.

Some new contexts, pictures, and scripts for situations the child finds challenging in real life (taken from the child's ISCP).

Procedure

Role-reversal

Following from USC Activity 2, engage the child in role-reversal asking him to describe social contexts by behaviour and language.

Start by asking the child to describe one context by expected behaviours, "Tell me what someone might do in one of these places".

For accurate descriptions, collect the cards as you work out the right context.

For incomplete descriptions, explain that you need more information and guide the child to provide matching actions, e.g., "Can I run around?", "Am I inside or outside?".

Repeat, using the same cards saying, "This time give me a clue what someone in the picture will say", and support as needed to generate language to match the context.

Repeat USC 2 or continue to provide scaffolding in this activity until the child can give examples of behaviour and language for all contexts.

Observe the child's performance on familiar, unfamiliar, and personally challenging contexts for signs of understanding about what language and behaviours match in each context.

SCIP Phase 1

USC 4

Introduction to understanding social context

Activity 4: Simple personal reflection

Purpose and target

To help the child understand his own experiences as simple social situations and begin the process of reflecting on his experiences through considering what was said and done.

Materials

A few recent *straightforward* events as related by child, family, or school staff, collected from recent communication or taken from the Individual Social Communication Profile.

Picture cards for use as prompts if required (e.g., Combimage by Schubi)

Procedure

Following from USC Activities 2 and 3, explain that we can think about what has happened in our own experiences in the same way.

Describe the task as 'thinking about something that has already happened' and draw a picture with figures to represent the child and the other people needed to reflect on the situation.

Add speech bubbles and text to illustrate the events.

Add feelings to faces and thought bubbles if appropriate.

Emphasise that this is a story about what 'has already happened'.

Encourage the child to add to the events and to write or draw as they wish.

Ask the following questions in order: "Where were you?", "What were you doing?", "What were you thinking about?", "What did you say?", "What were you feeling?", "What did you want?".

Repeat these questions for the others in the event and discuss the events as fully as possible.

Explain that this is important because as you work together you will be thinking about 'things that have already happened' and about 'things that will happen soon', and that talking like this can help the child with feeling more comfortable and less worried/confused.

Be alert to the child's level of self-awareness and comfort and avoid probing for detail or dwelling on any context or event which is upsetting at this point. Examples can be added to the child's ISCP and Phase 2 planner for more detailed discussion and generating solutions in Phase 2 work.

SCIP Phase 1

MPA 1

Basic metapragmatic awareness

Activity 1: Listening for content

Purpose and target

To help the child develop the concept of actively listening to words; to develop heightened awareness of skills needed to enhance listening to the content of spoken language.

Materials

Puppet with large ears (or stick on some large ears temporarily).

Stories with several repetitions of key words (e.g., *Room on the Broom* by Julia Donaldson).

Cards with key words or symbols from the story. Include words that are frequent and infrequent and early and later in the texts.

Blank card to make a chart of listening skills with five columns and two rows marked out.

Procedure

Stick the ears on the puppet or draw attention to his big ears to explain, "We are going to teach the puppet how to listen to the words".

Show the target words and say these are the words we are listening for in our story.

Select one that is mentioned early in the story to demonstrate the task.

Ask the puppet to put his hand up every time he hears the target word, e.g., 'cat'.

Ask the child to help the puppet listen for the word 'cat'.

Read the story aloud and pause after the first reading of the target word to allow the child to put the puppet's hand up.

Each time the child correctly hears the word and responds with his/puppet's hand up stop to discuss what helped to hear the target word, e.g., thinking about the words, looking at the speaker, not fidgeting/sitting still, etc.

Add a symbol or word to the child's chart of listening skills for the listening behaviours used.

Each time the word appears and is identified add a smiley face to the chart under these listening behaviours and emphasise the phrase "listening and thinking about the words".

Repeat with a new word from the story and continue to emphasise the link between success on the task and the listening behaviours.

Each time the child hears the selected word, add a smile under the skills you wish to reinforce and make sure the child and the puppet get some rewards each.

By the end of the activity, the chart should contain skills such as thinking about the words, looking at the speaker, knowing what was said, asking for help.

Meta-challenge

Gradually extend the length of time the child needs to wait to hear the key word in the story by choosing less frequent words. Introduce interruptions and explain that it is harder to listen and think about the words when it is noisy or after an interruption or distraction. Call this 'thinking about something else'.

SCIP Phase 1

MPA 2

Basic metapragmatic awareness

Activity 2: Understanding behaviours associated with listening

Purpose and target

To develop the child's understanding of the impact of different behaviours on active listening and to develop a heightened awareness of how to use active listening strategies.

Materials

New puppet with little ears (to signify poor listening).

Stories with repeated words similar to that used in MPA 1.

Examples of listening skills the child needs to learn from the ISCP.

The child's chart of listening skills from MPA 1.

Procedure

Following from MPA 1, repeat the listening activity with a new story, but this time explain that we need to teach the new puppet to listen well.

Meta-challenge

Start the story and make the new puppet engage in each of the following behaviours one by one:

- ❖ not sitting still
- ❖ looking around
- ❖ picking up objects and having a look at them
- ❖ putting his hand up for the wrong word
- ❖ talking at the same time

In sequence, make the puppet do each of these behaviours so that the child misses the key word he should be listening for. Stop the story after each occurrence of the word and ask the child to give the puppet some advice so that it can actively listen for the key word.

Make it clear that the puppet hasn't been able to listen to the key words and win smiles on its chart because it has been fidgeting, looking away, or talking at the same time, etc.

Emphasise the phrase "not listening and not thinking about the words".

Emphasise the link between success on the task and the listening behaviours, e.g., "If he wants to think about the words, he needs to stop talking at the same time".

Repeat for all behaviours and another target word.

Make sure that you have included skills the child wants to improve, e.g., interrupting or thinking about something else.

Revise by reviewing the chart of the behaviours that help us to listen, including *thinking about the story/words*, *not talking at the same time*, etc.

Repeat once more with a new story and new target words and ask the child to show the puppet how to listen well. As the child hears each target word, add a smile to the chart under the identified behaviours, paying special attention to any the child wants to practise. Emphasise skills used by the child and the link with success on the task.

SCIP Phase 1

MPA 3

Basic metapragmatic awareness

Activity 3: Developing metapragmatic vocabulary

Purpose and target

To help the child understand the characteristics of a speaker and listener and develop the vocabulary needed to describe the speaker and listener roles in conversation.

Materials

Two A4 pages, pencils, and coloured pencils.
Chart created in MPA 1 (as prompt, only if needed).

Procedure

Explain the task as making posters of a listener and a speaker. Start with a 'good listening' poster as this has just been covered in MPA Activity 2, but extend the ideas to include what is needed in conversation.

Ask the child to draw a face with big ears and label this the 'listener' to get the poster started.

Ask the child to think of all the things that good listeners do when they are listening to their friends and write these on the poster.

Encourage the child to draw pictures and add his own words for listening. Add additional words and ideas as necessary.

To draw a poster of a speaker, ask the child to draw a face with a big mouth and label this the 'speaker'.

Add skills listed below and discuss as much as possible with the child.

Add any other skills that the child needs to become more aware of and practise from his ISCP.

Listener

- ❖ listening to others' ideas
- ❖ not talking at the same time
- ❖ no interrupting
- ❖ no changing the subject
- ❖ wait for my turn
- ❖ looking at the other person

Speaker

- ❖ looking at the other person
- ❖ say something in return about the ideas
- ❖ wait for a response
- ❖ stay on the same subject
- ❖ answer questions

SCIP Phase 1
MPA 4
Basic metapragmatic awareness
Activity 4: Listener–speaker role-play

Purpose and target

To develop the child's awareness of speaker and listener characteristics and ability to describe the speaker and listener roles using learned metapragmatic vocabulary.

Materials

Picture cards showing a familiar scene with at least two people who could be having an imagined conversation (e.g., shop, doctor's surgery, family scene).

Speech bubble cards or sticky notes.

Speaker and listener rules on cards (as created in MPA 3).

Chart created in MPA 1.

Procedure

Role-play

Explain that it's time to practise being a listener and speaker and refer to the posters from MPA Activity 3.

Present one picture card and explain the location and topic for a short conversation between the characters.

Choose one role for yourself and allocate one for the child.

Role-play one short exchange between the people in the picture and stop.

Refer explicitly to the listening and speaking skills used and award smiles to each person as reinforcement, e.g., "I asked you a question and you listened to the question and then gave me an answer. That is being a good listener and a good speaker".

Repeat and try to extend the exchange.

Use the skill cards to give feedback to each other.

Add new skills to the posters as they occur in the conversation, e.g., 'answer questions'.

Emphasise that the conversation was working well because the speaker and listener were using skills of speaking and listening to each other.

Discuss how you could tell that an answer was needed, e.g., "You asked me what I wanted so I needed to tell you my answer".

Repeat with a new scene until all skills have been practised.

Review the posters at the end in a general discussion of skills needed and used, add any new skills coming from the activity and the discussion.

SCIP Phase 1

BN 1

Basic narrative

Activity 1: Understanding vocabulary for sequencing

Purpose and target

To develop the child's understanding of vocabulary required to support picture sequencing: first, next, last, before, and after.

Materials

Playmobil (or similar small people toys) scene and people.

Black Sheep Press 2-step sequence pictures or similar.

Black Sheep Press Before/After and First/Next/Last worksheets or similar.

Procedure

Role-play

Using the Playmobil, set up a scene that requires three or four people to form a queue for an event or activity, e.g., a slide or swing, or an ice cream seller.

Describe each person's position in the queue as first/next/last.

Role-play the first person moving forward and receiving her/his turn.

Repeat the words 'first', 'next', and 'last' often and repeat with different events until the child is beginning to join in and name the positions.

To check that the child understands these words, ask him to point to each position in the queue.

Role-reversal

Ask the child to control the scene and set up a new queue for a different event.

Ask the child to explain what is happening as he moves the people through the queue to the event.

Set up larger scenes to act out completing a list of events in order, e.g., "First I want to have an ice cream, next I want to watch the dolphins, and last I want to take a photograph".

Ask the child to move the character around the scene in order to your instruction.

Role-reversal

Ask the child to tell you what activities to do first/next/last.

Repeat this activity using the words 'before' and 'after' if needed or use the words 'before' and 'after' in your descriptions if this is not confusing for the child.

Use the 2-step picture sets or simple story books to teach the words 'before' and 'after' if needed.

SCIP Phase 1

BN 2

Basic narrative

Activity 2: Making simple inferences from pictures

Purpose and target

To help the child make simple inferences from pictures that support making predictions of what could/did happen in a sequence of pictures.

Materials

Selected materials from *Introducing Inference* by Marilyn Toomey or similar.

'What happened next?' sets (picture 1 from a set of 3 sequence pictures).

'What is probably going to happen?' sets (pictures 1 and 2 from a set of 3).

'What probably happened?' sets (picture 1 and 3 from a set of 3 sequence sets).

Procedure

Introduce the task as looking at some stories together and working out what is going to happen next by looking for clues in the pictures.

Show the child the first picture from the first set of 'What happened next?' items and say, "Let's talk about what is happening here".

Talk about the two pictures and then say, "What do you think is going to happen?".

If the child can't think of anything, provide him with some alternatives and ask him to select one.

If the child quickly answers the question of what happens next, then ask, "How do you know that?".

Make explicit reference to the clues in the pictures and draw circles around the salient points in each to demonstrate that the clues to working things out are in the picture, e.g., "I know that the girl must have dropped the eggs because here she is holding them and here, they are on the floor all broken".

Emphasise the link between the important information in the pictures and how it supports the inferences made.

Emphasise vocabulary taught in CM 2, i.e., working out and not guessing.

Give explanations and generalisations of predicable consequences, e.g., "That usually happens like that".

Discuss additional inferences that can be made from the scenes depicted such as feelings, solutions to problems, etc.

SCIP Phase 1

BN 3

Basic narrative

Activity 3: Simple sequencing

Purpose and target

To help the child understand event sequences; to be able to arrange up to four pictures in order and describe events in the sequence.

Materials

Winslow Press 4-step sequence cards, Black Sheep Press 3 and 4-step sequences, or similar.
Traditional stories sequence sets.
Blank card/Question mark card.

Procedure

Model one sequence of a familiar event by setting out the first in sequence and making inferences, as in BN2. Show the next card in the sequence to demonstrate that the inference was correct. Repeat with working out the third and fourth scenes until all cards in the sequence have been laid out.

Now, describe the sequence using simple sentences for each picture, and include information on who is in the story, what happens, and the location.

Discuss and explain explicitly what will probably happen next [prediction].

Clearly explain any reasons you have for the prediction or for the event sequence described [inference].

Emphasise the link between the important information in each of the pictures and how it supports the inferences and predictions made.

Repeat with a new sequence set and ask the child to join in with describing and making inferences. Continue to emphasise the link between the important information in each of the pictures and how it supports the inferences made.

Gradually give the child a full set to sequence and encourage the child to set out each picture in order by using inferences to determine the order and giving reasons for the decisions.

Support him to gain all the information he can from one picture as the starting point, before looking at all pictures together.

Ask the child to describe the complete sequence using language to reflect the inferences, e.g., "I know he's going to the park to play on his skateboard because he is carrying his skateboard and the sign says 'Park'".

Add a question mark card at any point in the sequence and ask the child to add an event that has been inferred but not shown.

Ask the child to draw an additional event on blank card to add detail before or after the existing sequence set.

SCIP Phase 1

BN 4

Basic narrative

Activity 4: Simple personal stories

Purpose and target

To help the child understand his own experiences as simple narratives and begin the process of reflecting on his experiences through retelling actual events.

Materials

Paper cut into quarters to act as single cards in a simple sequenced story.

Recent events (without challenges) as related by child, family, or school staff, collected from recent communication or taken from the ISCP.

Picture cards for use as prompts if required (e.g., Winslow Resources Tell Me About It; GLS Learning to sequence 4 Scene sets).

Procedure

Describe the task as drawing a story about something that has really happened and draw a simple three-step story about your own recent experience, e.g., drive to school, sign in at the office, come to class to collect the child.

Add speech bubbles and text to illustrate the events.

Add feelings to faces and thought bubbles if useful.

Add a final picture of you and the child working together in the room you are in.

Emphasise that this is a story about what has already happened.

Ask the child to remember a simple unproblematic event from their week and prompt as necessary from what you have heard from parents and teacher.

Draw or help the child to draw the sequence starting with first event.

Add speech bubbles and text to illustrate the events.

Add feelings to faces and thought bubbles if useful.

Discuss with the child what happened next and continue for two more pictures making explicit reference to all the events and inferences that can be made from the story as in BN2.

Support the child to describe the sequence explicitly using his own words and ideas and perceptions of the event.

SCIP Phase 1

EM 1

Introduction to emotions in context

Activity 1: Matching pictures and symbols to facial expressions

Purpose and target

To develop the child's understanding of vocabulary, symbols, and facial expressions for four emotions (happy/sad/afraid/angry).

Materials

Pairs of photos of facial expressions to represent each of the four emotions, e.g., Emotions Fun Deck or similar.

Pairs of symbols of happy, sad, afraid, and angry.

Mirror.

Procedure

Lay out one photo of each emotion and hold the matching set of photos in your hand.

Mime one at a time and ask the child to "Point to the one I am doing".

If he is correct, give the matching card to the child.

Repeat with all four photos until the child has 'won' them all.

Revise any that the child is unsure of before repeating this task using the symbols to ensure the child can recognise simple line drawings of facial expressions which will be used in later sessions.

Role-reversal

Engage the child in role-reversal by giving them a set of photos and asking them to make a face to match the emotion for you to choose from the photos laid out.

Observe the child's ability to mimic facial expressions.

In discussion, ask for words or events that accompany each emotion and if useful talk to the child about recent times when they or someone they know has experienced each emotion and record these examples on the ISCP.

SCIP Phase 1

EM 2

Introduction to emotions in context

Activity 2: Linking emotions to events

Purpose and target

To help the child understand the relationship between events and emotions in simple social situations.

Materials

Single pictures of social contexts depicting each of the feelings in Activity 1, e.g., Schubi/ Westerman Sentimage or Black Sheep Press Practical Pragmatics, or similar.

Speech bubble sticky notes.

Procedure

Using a scene that represents a happy event, say that the task is to work out how the people feel by looking for clues in the pictures.

Describe the picture making explicit reference to the reasons for the description as in BN2, e.g., "This girl has won a prize. She will say, 'Great, I won!' She will think, 'I am lucky today'. She will be smiling and laughing; she feels happy".

Ask the child to write the person's words into the speech bubble by asking, "What will she say?".

Create a thought bubble and ask, "What will she be thinking?".

Ask the child to draw the facial expression and write the emotion word underneath.

Personalisation

Ask for an example of what makes the child you are working with feel happy and make a drawing of this. Add this to the ISCP.

Repeat for the feelings sad, scared, and angry. For emotions other than happy/excited include some discussion of possible solutions by asking, "What would make it feel better? What could he do to help?".

SCIP Phase 1

EM 3

Introduction to emotions in context

Activity 3: Emotions Ladder

Purpose and target

To help the child understand that feelings change in relation to events experienced and to create a visual representation of how feelings change.

Materials

Four ladders with at least three rungs drawn on an A4 sheet of paper (landscape).
Four events taken from EM2, one for each feeling, happy/sad/angry/scared.
Coloured pens or pencils.
Symbols, photos, or words to represent emotions.

Procedure

Following from EM Activity 2, discuss that the task is to create a ladder of feelings to show that feelings can change.

Start with happy and ask the child to choose a colour to represent happy feelings.

Write the word 'Happy' as a heading for the first ladder on the page.

Write 'OK' at the bottom of this ladder and 'Happy' at the top.

Between the words 'OK' and 'Happy' write or stick a picture of an event that would make someone feel happy (use examples from Activity 2).

Draw an arrow upwards from 'OK' to 'Happy' and explain that, e.g., when the girl wins a prize, her feelings change from OK to Happy. Emphasise the link between the event and the change in her feelings, e.g., before she won, she felt OK, after she won, she felt happy, etc.

Encourage the child to illustrate the ladder with drawings of happy faces and anything that represents the example used, e.g., a trophy.

Repeat for each feeling using the child's choice of colour for each feeling, adding symbols and/or words that will be useful for the child.

Discuss additional events that may lead to each of these feelings in general terms.

Personalisation

Using information on the child's feelings from the ISCP, or from discussion in EM2, draw a ladder to represent a change from feeling OK to Happy and engage the child in writing and drawing, as above. Do not engage in discussion of other emotions at this stage, but, if the child volunteers information, add it to the ISCP.

SCIP Phase 1

EM 4

Introduction to emotions in context

Activity 4: Making inferences from facial expression and direction of eye gaze

Purpose and target

To help the child understand that non-verbal behaviour, such as eye gaze and facial expression, carry social meanings related to others' thoughts and intentions.

Materials

Two puppets.
Miniature objects, e.g., cake/dustpan/books/post box/keys/pen.

Procedure

Arrange up to four objects at intervals around the table.

Ask the child to work out which thing your puppet wants to play with by watching what it is doing.

Make your puppet look at the thing it wants; exaggerate as required.

Discuss by stating, "You worked out what he wanted by following his eyes". Explain in terms suitable to the child's comprehension.

Emphasise the link between the puppet's eye gaze and its thoughts, e.g., "I know he wants to play with the bus because he is looking at it", "If he wants to play with the bus, he will look at it".

Draw a picture of the puppet looking at the item and draw a line from the puppet's eyes to the item and a thinking bubble containing the item or the phrase, 'I want the ...'.

Ask the child to work his puppet to show what it would like to play with for you to work out.

Emphasise how you worked it out by following what the puppet was looking at.

Repeat with different objects, but this time, ask the child to watch you for a clue as to which items you like and those you don't like.

Look at one item and use clear facial expression to indicate like and dislike.

Draw the child's attention to the added meaning of the facial expression, "I am looking at it, but my face is saying 'I don't like it'. This means I don't want to play with it".

Draw an image to represent all three elements of eye gaze, facial expression, and item, and explain that sometimes people do this when they are playing together or talking.

Role-reversal

For children who are comfortable making eye contact, ask him to look at his choice without speaking to see if you can work it out. Use phrases such as, "I know you are interested in the post box because you are looking at it".

If the child is happy to try to use facial expression to signal 'I want' and 'I don't want', model again and engage in role-reversal. Explain that even though he didn't say anything, you could work it out because you could see what he was looking at and could see his facial expression, which worked to send the message. Use the room you are in and look at items for the child to work out what you like and what you don't like.

Phase 1 to Phase 2 Pointers

The Phase 1 Pointer content table below shows one activity for each of the Phase 1 Components. Each activity states its required materials, some of which may have been used or created during Phase 1 delivery.

Phase 1 to Phase 2 Pointer content table

Phase 1 Component	Phase 1 Pointer activities
Comprehension monitoring (CM)	Demonstrating the ability to monitor comprehension and actively seek clarification
Introduction to understanding social context (USC)	Demonstrating the ability to match behaviour and language to a range of social situations
Basic metapragmatic awareness (BMA)	Demonstrating the ability to listen in conversation
Basic narrative (BN)	Demonstrating the ability to sequence sets of pictures and tell a simple story in order
Introduction to emotions in context (EM)	Demonstrating the ability to match feelings to context

SCIP Phase 1

CM Pointer

Comprehension monitoring

Demonstrating the ability to monitor comprehension and actively and appropriately seek clarification

Purpose and target

To heighten the child's awareness of what he usually does when he is confused. To enable the child to identify when he is unsure of what to do. To encourage the child to make confident and appropriate requests for clarification while engaged in a high-interest activity.

Materials

Construction game/making an object or game which involves giving instructions such as making a paper aeroplane or reusable sticker scene sets.

Prepare in advance a set of easy and complicated or confusing instructions.

Child's record of comprehension monitoring strategies from CM3.

Procedure

Explain to child that you are going to give him instructions that will help him complete the chosen task.

Start by giving a straightforward instruction.

At intervals, give an impossible or confusing instruction.

Observe the child's reaction to these instructions, pause and allow time for him to use a request for clarification.

Avoid causing anxiety and prompt to use strategies for clarification as needed.

Input guidance

Observe the child's level of awareness of being confused and his preferred way of requesting clarification. Decide what consolidation is required in terms of comprehension monitoring and add this to the Phase 2 Planner. Observe the child's non-verbal behaviours and any signs of confusion that he is spontaneously using. Document these and make explicit reference to them with the child so that he is increasingly self-aware. Observe any unhelpful compensation behaviours that the child is using when he is confused and record these on the Phase 2 Planner. Share with staff for support in class.

SCIP Phase 1

USC Pointer

Introduction to understanding social context

Demonstrating the ability to match behaviour and language to a range of social situations

Purpose and target

To heighten the child's awareness of how spoken language and behaviour relate to the context/situation. To enable the child to identify a social context from either the language used or a description of the behaviours. To enable the child to begin to reflect on his own behaviour and language in social situations.

Materials

Set of social context pictures, some familiar and some unfamiliar.

Include some that match the situations that the child finds difficult as reported by parents and teachers from the child's ISCP, e.g., running around the supermarket.

Descriptions of language typically used in each context.

Descriptions of behaviours seen in each context.

Procedure

Lay out one context and the matching language and behaviour cards.

Show that the descriptions match the picture.

Explain that the task is to play a pairs game by matching the descriptions to the pictures.

Lay out a selection of contexts, behaviours, and language, so as to be able to make a game but without using so many that the child is overwhelmed.

Take turns selecting one card from each group and see if they match.

Discuss each picture as it is turned over, e.g., after selecting a behaviour card ask what context the child is looking for and what language he might expect.

Read descriptions aloud if necessary and discuss with the child.

Keep any pairs and play until all cards are matched, adding new sets as existing ones are matched.

Input guidance

Observe the child's awareness of the link between language to behaviour, language to context, and context to behaviour. Observe how his knowledge reflects his actual behaviours in real life situations, e.g., does he know that talking does not match the school Assembly context, but still persist in talking in Assembly? Decide what consolidation is required in terms of self-awareness and self-monitoring. Add this to the Phase 2 Planner. Observe the child's response to being confused and add this to information on comprehension monitoring.

SCIP Phase 1

MPA Pointer

Basic metapragmatic awareness

Demonstrating the ability to listen in conversation

Purpose and target

To observe the child's ability to use active listening skills taught in Phase 1 and to determine the need for continued support in Phase 2.

Materials

Symbol chart of listening skills developed in Phase 1.

Suitable prop or picture to create a topic of conversation.

Procedure

Show the child the picture or object that will act as a conversation topic and begin to talk to him about it. Get him involved in the conversation and observe how he listens and responds in line with previous Phase 1 goals.

Stop the conversation and ask the child to think about what speaker and listener skills he used. Start him off by saying, "Let's have a think about how well you used your listening skills when we were talking. I could see that you were listening because you were answering my questions". Ask the child to mark a smile on his chart under these skills.

Ask the child to comment on what he was trying to do and observe what words he uses to describe himself and how accurate he is in judging his performance.

Give some feedback on what he did well and what he still needs to work at and make a note on the Phase 2 Planner of how to support independent monitoring of listening skills.

Input guidance

This activity can be repeated at intervals throughout Phase 2 to build the child's self-awareness and ability to self-monitor listening skills in conversation. Additional skills can be added at intervals to the chart as intervention progresses.

SCIP Phase 1

BN Pointer

Basic narrative

Demonstrating the ability to sequence sets of pictures and tell a simple story in order

Purpose and target

To observe the child's ability to organise a series of up to six pictures into a coherent sequence of events. To enable the child to develop his ability to make inferences from pictures, commenting on the relatedness and relevance of specific events in given narratives.

Materials

6–8 step sequence sets from Winslow Press or Schubi Tell Me About It.
Blank cards to act as gaps in the stories.

Procedure

Explain to the child that this task is helping each other to put the picture sequences into order.

Take the first turn and arrange one sequence set with at least one card in the wrong place. Observe if the child can find the error and explain why it is wrong.

Tell the story as it is laid out and observe the child's ability to correct the error.

When you get to the error, discuss the details in the pictures surrounding the error and how this helps to repair the error.

Ask the child to take a turn setting out the pictures to tell a story and observe his ability to use information in the pictures to decide the order of events.

For all sets, present some blank cards and ask the child to fill in the gaps by discussing what else could happen at the end or the beginning.

Input guidance

Observe the child's ability to recognise the error and what information he is not able to detect from each picture. Decide what consolidation is required in terms of understanding narrative and add this to the Phase 2 Planner. Observe the child's response to being confused and add this to information on Phase 2 comprehension monitoring.

SCIP Phase 1

EM Pointer

Introduction to emotions in context

Demonstrating the ability to match feelings to context

Purpose and target

To heighten the child's awareness that there are expected feelings for given situations and provide information on the child's needs for intervention in Phase 2.

Materials

Black Sheep Press Practical Pragmatics or Sentimage cards from Schubi.

Set of matching facial expressions and events for feelings to include happy, sad, angry, and scared.

Procedure

Lay out one context and the matching facial expression card.

Discuss that the feeling matches the picture and make reference to the child's own experiences of this feeling.

Explain that the task is to play a pairs game by matching the feelings to the pictures.

Lay out a selection of contexts and facial expressions, so as to be able to make a game but without using so many that the child is overwhelmed.

Take turns selecting one card from each group and see if they match.

Discuss each picture as it is turned over, e.g., after selecting a context card, ask what feeling the child is looking for and vice versa.

Keep any pairs and play until all cards are matched, adding new sets as existing ones are matched.

Ensure resources are used for each feeling that has been practised in Phase 1.

Use written words and symbols as appropriate to the child.

Input guidance

Observe the child's awareness of the match of feelings to contexts. Decide what consolidation is required in terms of understanding emotions in context and add this to the Phase 2 Planner. Observe the child's response to being confused and add this to information on comprehension monitoring.

SCIP Assessment to Intervention Map

The Phase 2 Assessment to Intervention Map provides guidance against which to judge the child's profile of need and to decide which Sections and Objectives are to be included in Phase 2 Planning.

SCIP Phase 2 Assessment to Intervention Map	
Social Understanding and Social Interpretation (SUSI)	
Section	**Guidance for inclusion in Phase 2**
SUSI 1 Understanding social context cues in interactions	Can misinterpret social situations; makes mismatched comments; may mismatch social cues within context
	Teacher report: Mismatched comments in social situations; needs in using language in specific context
	Parent report: Sometimes seems as if he doesn't know what to say or ask for
SUSI 2 Understanding emotion cues in interactions	Has needs in understanding and expressing emotions in context; may not recognise non-verbal cues
	CCC-2: "Looks blank in a situation where most children would show a clear facial expression; fails to recognise when others are upset or angry"
	Parent report: Can be unaware of others' feelings
	Practitioner: Limited emotion vocabulary use in Phase 1
SUSI 3 Understanding and practising flexibility	Prefers routine and sameness; change needs to be carefully managed; unplanned change is upsetting
	Parent report: I have to do the same things in the same order, or he gets very upset
	CCC-2: "Chooses the same favourite activity"
	Teacher report: He sometimes won't start work until everyone is sitting down; he sometimes tells other children what to do
SUSI 4 Understanding thoughts and intentions of others	Challenges in making verbal or social inferences; does not understand deception, tricks, or jokes; makes unintentionally hurtful comments
	Parent report: Sometimes he says very embarrassing things to people. I worry that he is too trusting
	CCC-2: "Misses the point of jokes or puns; Hurts or upsets others without meaning to"
	Teacher report: He doesn't understand tricks or jokes with peers, gets easily upset in games and withdraws
SUSI 5 Understanding friendship	Finds it hard to join in with peer group; isolated in playground, watches others but does not approach anyone
	Parent/teacher report: He wants a friend very badly but is often left out
	CCC-2: "Appears anxious in the company of other children; is left out of joint activities"
	Practitioner: Playground observation showed limited interactions with peers in social time

SCIP Phase 2 Assessment to Intervention Map	
Pragmatics	
Section	**Guidance for inclusion in Phase 2**
PRAG 1 Turn-taking and reciprocity	Does not relinquish or take up turns in conversation; has needs in reciprocity and turn-taking
	TOPICC: Lack of reciprocity in conversation. It is hard to interrupt the child's flow of talk
	Parent report: He is inconsistent in conversation, sometimes ignores me, sometimes talks over me
	CCC-2: "Ignores conversational overtures from others"
PRAG 2 Conversation and metapragmatic skills	Conversational flow shows some misunderstandings which the child cannot clarify; may not initiate or ask questions; may not recognise non-verbal signals to start or stop talking
	TOPICC: No initiation in conversation probes
	Parent report: He does not ask any questions even if it is something he is interested in, he will remain silent. I can see that he has misinterpreted something, but he doesn't notice
	CCC-2: "Ignores conversational overtures from others"
PRAG 3 Understanding information requirements	Includes very precise information but also talks about things either not established or already known; referents are sometimes unclear
	CCC-2: "Doesn't explain what he is talking about to someone who doesn't share his experiences"
	Parent report: It can be very hard to follow his ideas in conversation; he stops me to correct or question me if he thinks I have been imprecise
PRAG 4 Understanding and managing topic in conversation	Preferred topics dominate conversation; unaware of others' level of interest; does not signal topic change; lists facts
	Parent report: Frequently changes topic in conversation to his interests, starts talking without letting us know what he is talking about, e.g., he might say, 'nothing is impossible'
	CCC-2: "Talks repetitively about things no-one is interested in; talks about lists of things he has memorised; moves the conversation to a favourite topic even though others don't seem interested"
PRAG 5 Understanding and improving discourse style	Changing style to match different types of interactions is challenging; can appear overly formal or familiar in conversation
	Parent report: Talks to unfamiliar people too readily and is generally too friendly

SCIP Phase 2 Assessment to Intervention Map	
Language processing	
Section	**Guidance for inclusion in Phase 2**
LP 1 Vocabulary and word knowledge	**Naming/receptive vocabulary test** scores outside the expected range or performance indicates word-finding needs.
	Parent report: He gets frustrated because he cannot find the right words to say
	CCC-2: "Forgets words he knows; is vague in choice of words; mixes up words of similar meaning"
	Teacher report: He mixes up words I know he knows, like saying lion for leopard; often starts his sentences two or three times and sometimes gives descriptions for words
	Practitioner: Narrative or conversation is interrupted by word searching or unusual word choices; evidence of neologisms or substitutions in word choices in narrative or conversation
LP 2 Narrative construction	**Narrative test** scores outside the expected range: ERRNI Recall; ACE Narrative subtest
	Parent report: I can't tell what he means when he tells me something
	CCC-2: "Gets the sequence of events muddled up; hard to make sense of what he is saying"
	Teacher report: He cannot construct a simple narrative in literacy lessons, verbally he can tell one part of the story at a time but with no overall sense of what the story is about
LP 3 Non-literal language	Inferential comprehension needs; understanding of similes, metaphors, homophones, and idioms shows characteristics associated with younger children
LP 4 Discourse comprehension	Has needs in comprehension of complex sentences, text, or conversation from formal testing or report of performance at home/school
	Scores outside the expected range on formal testing of comprehension of complex sentences, text, or conversation, e.g., ACE: Inferential Comprehension; Sentence Comprehension
	TOPICC: Child cannot follow thread of conversation
	Teacher report: Frequently fails to understand; needs simplification of instructions in lessons
LP 5 Enhanced comprehension monitoring	Practitioner observations from Phase 1 comprehension monitoring sessions indicate need for further work
	Parent/teacher report: Often misunderstands but carries on without checking; he needs someone to point out that he has made a mistake or misunderstood; guesses at what he should be doing in class

PHASE 2 RESOURCE

Phase 2 Intervention content table

The Phase 2 Intervention content table provides an *overview* of the content of Phase 2 in its entirety. The three Phase 2 Components are arranged in three columns, Social Understanding and Social Interpretation (SUSI), Pragmatics (PRAG), and Language Processing (LP). Each box in the Phase 2 Intervention content table shows the Section for that Component.

The expanded content table showing all Sections and Objectives is also shown.

The nested structure of Phase 2 Intervention is provided as a reminder.

To access the Section intervention content, turn to the Section content tables on the relevant page. The intervention activities for that Section will follow directly after the Section content table.

Phase 2 Intervention Content Table: Components and Sections

Phase 2 Intervention content table		
Social Understanding and Social Interpretation (SUSI)	*Pragmatics (PRAG)*	*Language Processing (LP)*
SUSI 1 Understanding social context cues in interactions	PRAG 1 Turn-taking and reciprocity	LP 1 Vocabulary and word knowledge
SUSI 2 Understanding emotion cues in interactions	PRAG 2 Conversation and metapragmatic skills	LP 2 Narrative construction
SUSI 3 Understanding and practising flexibility	PRAG 3 Understanding information requirements	LP 3 Non-literal language
SUSI 4 Understanding thoughts and intentions of others	PRAG 4 Understanding and managing topic in conversation	LP 4 Discourse comprehension
SUSI 5 Understanding friendship	PRAG 5 Understanding and improving discourse style	LP 5 Enhanced comprehension monitoring

DOI: 10.4324/9781032706641-3

Expanded Phase 2 Intervention content table (Sections and Objectives across the three Phase 2 Components)

SUSI	PRAG	LP
SUSI 1 Understanding social context cues in interactions	**PRAG 1 Turn-taking and reciprocity**	**LP 1 Vocabulary and word knowledge**
SUSI 1.1 Understanding non-verbal cues in context	PRAG 1.1 Understanding how to take turns	LP 1.1 Understanding semantic relationships between words
SUSI 1.2 Strategies for problem solving in simple social contexts	PRAG 1.2 Understanding verbal turn-taking	LP 1.2 Consolidation and self-cueing
SUSI 2 Understanding emotion cues in interactions	PRAG 1.3 Consolidating turn-taking skills	LP 1.3 Vocabulary enrichment
SUSI 2.1 Building emotion vocabulary	**PRAG 2 Conversation and metapragmatic skills**	**LP 2 Narrative construction**
SUSI 2.2 Enhanced emotion vocabulary	PRAG 2.1 Enhanced listening skills	LP 2.1 Understanding inferences in picture sequences
SUSI 2.3 Understanding complex feelings	PRAG 2.2 Understanding speaker roles	LP 2.2 Telling complex and personalised stories
SUSI 3 Understanding and practising flexibility	PRAG 2.3 Giving information	LP 2.3 Constructing novel stories with plots
SUSI 3.1 Understanding routines	PRAG 2.4 Developing metapragmatic awareness	**LP 3 Non-literal language**
SUSI 3.2 Understanding and coping with unplanned change	**PRAG 3 Understanding information requirements**	LP 3.1 Understanding homophones
SUSI 3.3 Making changes in personal routines	PRAG 3.1 Understanding impact of missing information	LP 3.2 Understanding literal and non-literal meanings
SUSI 4 Understanding thoughts and intentions of others	PRAG 3.2 Understanding impact of too much information	LP 3.3 Understanding non-literal meanings in context
SUSI 4.1 Signalling feelings and intentions (non-verbal)	PRAG 3.3 Understanding matching context and talk	**LP 4 Discourse comprehension**
SUSI 4.2 Predicting thoughts and intentions	PRAG 3.4 Understanding information requirements in personal conversation	LP 4.1 Improving memory and listening
SUSI 4.3 Understanding mismatch of language and thoughts	**PRAG 4 Understanding and managing topic in conversation**	LP 4.2 Understanding verbal inferences
SUSI 4.4 Understanding complex intentions	PRAG 4.1 Identifying topics	LP 4.3 Understanding stories
SUSI 5 Understanding friendship	PRAG 4.2 Understanding topic change conventions	**LP 5 Enhanced comprehension monitoring**
SUSI 5.1 Understanding interests in friendship	PRAG 4.3 Consolidating topic skills	LP 5.1 Text level comprehension monitoring
SUSI 5.2 Understanding the impact of preferred interests	**PRAG 5 Understanding and improving discourse style**	LP 5.2 Task based comprehension monitoring
SUSI 5.3 Understanding friendship skills	PRAG 5.1 Understanding different styles in interaction	
	PRAG 5.2 Understanding and using conventions of interaction style	
	PRAG 5.3 Consolidating interaction style	

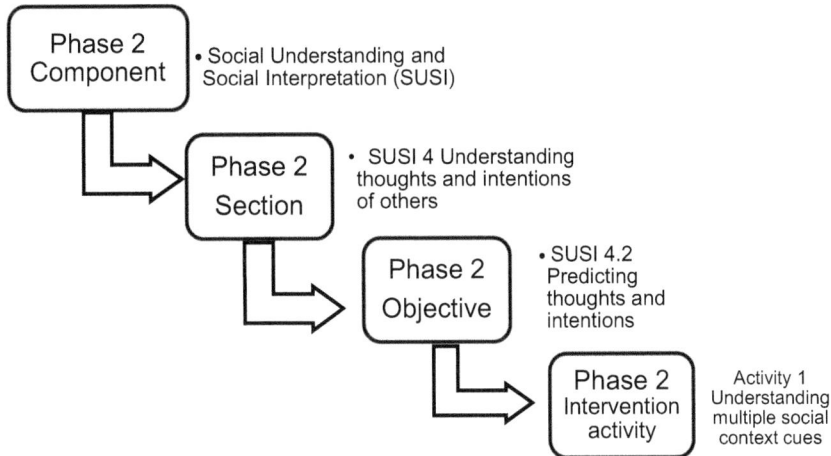

The nested structure of Phase 2 Intervention

Quick guide: List of activity targets in SUSI, PRAG, and LP
SUSI 1 Understanding social context cues in interactions
SUSI 1.1 Understanding non-verbal cues in context

1. to help the child understand how eye gaze can signal an intention. The child will be able to use eye gaze as a non-verbal means of communicating basic social intentions to other people
2. to help the child understand how to recognise cues in the social context in order to read social meanings
3. to support the child to be able to identify and describe expected future events, emotions, and thoughts for recent personal experiences

SUSI 1.2 Strategies for problem-solving in simple social communication contexts

1. to help the child identify that simple problems can be easily fixed and be able to generate possible solutions to given social scenarios
2. to introduce the child to the idea that he can resolve simple problems in his own experiences

SUSI 2 Understanding emotion cues in interactions
SUSI 2.1 Building emotion vocabulary

1. the child will be able to identify expected emotions for simple social contexts and describe a social situation that would give rise to a specified emotion

2. to help the child understand that feelings differ in intensity and to learn words to express these differing intensities using a visual representation for support
3. to help the child understand that feelings differ in intensity depending on the event and what it means to each person
4. to help the child understand the idea of over-reactions to events and that emotion reactions usually match the event

SUSI 2.2 Enhanced emotion vocabulary

1. to help the child understand that emotions can be conceptualised and described in abstract terms and through images
2. to help the child use idioms to describe emotions as a way of conceptualising and describing emotions in abstract terms

SUSI 2.3 Understanding complex feelings

1. to help the child identify expected emotions for a range of social contexts. To enable the child to describe a social situation that would give rise to a specified emotion
2. to facilitate the child's understanding of matching emotions for complex social situations; to help the child describe expected emotions, thoughts, and words for complex social contexts
3. to facilitate the child's understanding of his own emotional reactions in complex social situations; to help the child to describe his own and others' perspectives and suggest solutions for emotional reactions

SUSI 3 Understanding and practising flexibility
SUSI 3.1 Understanding routines

1. to help the child understand vocabulary and concepts to describe routines and expectations associated with routines in order to enable him to understand and manage changes in routines
2. to help the child understand vocabulary and concepts to describe routines and expectations associated with the school day in order to enable him to understand and manage changes in routines
3. to help the child understand vocabulary and concepts to describe routines and expectations associated with the home routine in order to enable him to understand and manage changes in routines

SUSI 3.2 Understanding unplanned change

1. to help the child understand vocabulary and concepts associated with accidents, making mistakes, and associated feelings
2. to help the child understand vocabulary and concepts to describe unplanned change
3. to help the child understand vocabulary and concepts to describe unplanned change in games and social interactions

SUSI 3.3 Making changes in personal routines

1. to help the child understand the impact of being flexible on his own and other people's thoughts and feelings; to help him to be able to reflect on his own flexibility
2. to help the child understand the impact of being flexible on his own and other people's thoughts and feelings; to help him to be able to reflect on his own flexibility when unplanned changes happen

SUSI 4 Understanding thoughts and intentions of others
SUSI 4.1 Signalling feelings and intentions (non-verbal)

1. to enhance the child's awareness of the social meanings carried by non-verbal behaviour such as eye gaze and body position
2. to enhance the child's awareness of the social meanings (boredom and interest) carried by non-verbal behaviour such as eye gaze, facial expression, and body position

SUSI 4.2 Predicting thoughts and intentions

1. to help the child to identify and describe expected future events, emotions, and thoughts for a variety of characters in complex social situations
2. to help the child to identify and describe expected future events, emotions and thoughts for recent personal experiences

SUSI 4.3 Understanding mismatch of language and thoughts

1. to help the child understand the concept of lies and the purpose they serve; to develop the child's understanding of and ability to manage complex personal situations
2. to help the child understand the concept of white lies and the purpose they serve in complex personal situations

SUSI 4.4 Understanding complex intentions

1. to help the child understand the concept of tricks and the mismatch between language and thought so that he develops strategies to cope with complex personal situations
2. to help the child understand the concept of persuasion and understand how to give good reasons for things he wants to happen

SUSI 5 Understanding friendship
SUSI 5.1 Understanding interests in friendship

1. to help the child understand the importance of shared interests and asking about people's interests in building friendships
2. to help the child understand the importance of shared interests and finding out about people's interests in building friendships
3. to help the child understand his own interests as part of understanding the nature of shared interests in friendship
4. to help the child understand how his interests overlap with others or not and how to discuss interests to plan an enjoyable playtime
5. to help the child understand the importance of joining in with activities not of his choosing and develop strategies to show an interest in others
6. to help the child understand the importance of shared interests and finding out about people's interests in building friendships; the child will be able to ask questions to find a shared interest and use this to play with others

SUSI 5.2 Understanding the impact of preferred interests

1. to help the child to understand what his own preferred interests are and the feelings and words associated with them
2. to help the child to understand the impact of his own preferred interests on friendship and loneliness and provide support to try new interests
3. to help the child to understand the impact of his preferred interests on joining in with friendship or family activities; to provide support by emphasising the language of joining in and compromise
4. to enhance the child's understanding of vocabulary and concepts linked to fantasy and reality and become aware of fantasy elements in his own conversation
5. to help the child to understand the impact of fantasy worlds on learning and friendship

SUSI 5.3 Understanding friendship skills

1. to enable the child to practise different friendship skills, consolidate understanding of interests in friendship, and to practice friendship role-plays

2. to enable the child to identify a range of different friendship problems and learn how to resolve issues such as sharing, accidents, and being left out
3. to enable the child to identify a range of different friendship problems and identify issues that occur in his own friendships
4. to provide an opportunity for the child to reflect his own friendships and what he wants in a friend. To demonstrate an understanding of shared interests and qualities that make a good friend

PRAG 1 Turn-taking and reciprocity
PRAG 1.1 Understanding how to take turns

1. to help the child to understand basic turn-taking rules and vocabulary in a game
2. to help the child to understand basic turn-taking rules and vocabulary in a structured verbal interaction

PRAG 1.2 Understanding verbal turn-taking

1. to help the child to understand the sequences of listener and speaker talk and develop metapragmatic awareness of reciprocity in conversation
2. to enable the child to modify a sequence of listener and speaker talk by paying attention to the meaning of each utterance and to facilitate metapragmatic awareness of reciprocity in conversation
3. to help the child to develop metapragmatic awareness of how he manages reciprocity in conversation and be able to signal this awareness in his own conversations
4. to help the child understand the impact of using and not using turn-taking rules in conversation
5. to enhance the child's understanding of subtle turn-taking cues in conversation

PRAG 1.3 Consolidating turn-taking skills

1. to help the child in consolidating turn-taking skills for conversation
2. to help the child to understand his own turn-taking skills and to consolidate turn-taking skills for conversation

PRAG 2 Conversation and metapragmatic skills
PRAG 2.1 Enhanced listening skills

1. to reinforce the child's metapragmatic awareness of his own listening skills and support him to become able to self-monitor
2. to reinforce the child's metapragmatic awareness of the role of looking when listening to a speaker and understand the consequences of not looking

PRAG 2.2 Understanding speaker roles

1. to help the child to construct wh- questions to gain information and to understand and answer wh- questions
2. to enhance the child's ability to construct yes/no questions to gain information and be able to understand and answer yes/no questions
3. to enhance the child's ability to ask useful questions in conversation
4. to help the child to develop metapragmatic awareness of the impact of multiple questions on the interaction and to understand that the function of asking questions is to obtain useful information

PRAG 2.3 Giving information

1. to enhance the child's ability to give clear messages and to develop metapragmatic awareness of how to simplify information for the listener
2. to help the child learn to respond to requests for explanations and to develop metapragmatic awareness of how to simplify information for the listener

PRAG 2.4 Developing metapragmatic awareness

1. to help the child to explicitly identify conventions in conversation, and to understand how to react when conventions go wrong
2. to help the child to explicitly identify the convention he uses in conversation, and to understand how to modify those conventions in his own conversation

PRAG 3 Understanding information requirements
PRAG 3.1 Understanding impact of missing information

1. to help the child to understand the concepts of a lot, enough, and not enough as an introduction to understanding the concept of information in talking
2. the child will understand the consequences of missing information on comprehension of the whole story
3. to help the child understand the impact of minimal answers on conversation
4. to help the child understand how requests for clarification can be used to ask for missing information
5. to help the child use yes/no questions to ask for clarification and check information

PRAG 3.2 Understanding impact of too much information

1. to help the child understand the consequences of giving a lot of information during conversational interactions

2. to help the child understand the consequences of giving a lot of information during a game-based interaction
3. to introduce the child to the metapragmatic concepts of giving long answers and saying just enough
4. to assist the child to understand the effects of asking many questions during an interaction

PRAG 3.3 Understanding matching context and talk

1. to help the child begin to understand the metapragmatic concept of matching what is said to the physical and language context
2. to help the child understand the impact of matched and mismatched information on comprehension (simple)
3. to help the child understand the impact of matching and mismatching information in speech acts
4. the child will understand the metapragmatic concept of what information is known to other people
5. to help the child to understand how to distinguish between matched and mismatched information in conversation

PRAG 3.4 Understanding information requirements in personal conversation

1. to help the child develop the metapragmatic ability to monitor his own use of matched and mismatched information in conversation and begin to self-correct

PRAG 4 Understanding and managing topic in conversation
PRAG 4.1 Identifying topics

1. to help the child be able to identify topics in stories, to understand that the 'topic' is 'what is being talked about', and to use the word topic in metapragmatic discussions
2. to help the child learn about the metapragmatic concept of a favourite (or preferred) topic as something people like to talk about a lot. The child will identify favourite topics for himself and others
3. to help the child learn the metapragmatic concept of talking about different topics. The child will learn how people can talk about different topics

PRAG 4.2 Understanding topic change conventions

1. to help the child to be aware of and use accepted topic change conventions
2. to help the child to learn how to identify when topic change rules are broken; and to develop awareness of his own use of topic change markers

PRAG 4.3 Consolidating topic skills

1. to help the child learn to identify mismatched topics in talk and the effect they have on interaction
2. to help the child establish metapragmatic awareness of his own use of topics in interaction and to be able to change these with personalised guidance

PRAG 5 Understanding and improving discourse style
PRAG 5.1 Understanding different styles in interaction

1. to help the child understand and identify features of conversational style such as politeness, formality, and proximity: adult interlocutors
2. to help the child understand and identify features of conversational style such as politeness, formality, and proximity: child interlocutors
3. to help the child become familiar with the features of conversational style for interacting differently with known and not-known people
4. to assist the child to develop awareness of how people speak to each other differently depending on who they are and to suit the social context they are in
5. to help the child develop awareness of how people use different styles of verbal interaction to match the relationship and the context

PRAG 5.2 Understanding and using conventions of interaction style

1. to help the child understand conventions associated with greetings linked to relationships and context
2. to help the child understand pragmatic conventions associated with invitations linked to relationships and context
3. to help the child understand pragmatic conventions associated with farewells linked to relationships and context
4. to help the child develop awareness of how people use indirect speech acts as a form of politeness
5. to help the child understand and practice using indirect speech acts and to develop the child's awareness of how people use indirect speech acts as a form of politeness

PRAG 5.3 Consolidating interaction style

1. to help the child develop awareness of the impact of mismatched interaction styles and develop alternative strategies
2. to help the child to develop awareness of the impact of his own use of mismatches in style

LP 1 Vocabulary and word knowledge
LP 1.1 Understanding semantic relationships between words

1. to help the child understand how words and items can be grouped into categories
2. to help the child understand that words and items in categories can be grouped into sub-categories
3. to help the child to understand that items in categories can be differentiated based on the salient features of each item (similarities and differences)
4. to help the child to understand that items in categories can be differentiated based on the function each item performs
5. to help the child to understand that category names, functions, and specific semantic features are the essential elements of accurate word definitions

LP 1.2 Consolidation and self-cueing

1. to assist the child to understand and use a word-learning framework to support development of word knowledge across categories
2. to consolidate the child's understanding that category names, functions, and specific semantic features are the essential elements of accurate word definitions
3. to help the child to use word knowledge to self-cue in conversation

LP 1.3 Vocabulary enrichment

1. to help the child understand that synonyms are two different words with similar meanings and to be able to use synonyms in speech and writing
2. to help the child understand that antonyms are two words with opposite meanings and to be able to use antonyms in speech and writing
3. to assist the child in understanding the steps to follow in looking up words in a dictionary

LP 2 Narrative construction
LP 2.1 Understanding inferences in picture sequences

1. to help the child to understand that details in picture sequences can be used to make inferences and predictions, and are needed for coherent narratives
2. to enable the child to make inferences from relevant detail in picture sequences and to use this information to create coherent narratives

LP 2.2 Telling complex and personalised stories

1. to help the child to further develop the ability to relate events and stories, listing key elements of the story from the following: Introduction, setting the scene, locations, characters, events, problems, feelings, resolutions, and conclusions
2. to help the child to further develop the ability to retell events and stories, listing key aspects of the story from the following elements: Introduction, setting the scene, locations, characters, events, problems, feelings, resolutions, and conclusions
3. to practise retelling stories and events that might typically happen in children's lives
4. to practise retelling recent events that have happened with detail and in the expected sequence

LP 2.3 Constructing novel stories with plot

1. to support the child to create a simple novel story from given elements
2. to help the child understand how to introduce a new character to a story and create a role for that character in the story
3. to help the child understand how to introduce a change of location to a story and to make this meaningful in the story
4. to help the child understand how to introduce a fantasy element into a story and to make this meaningful in the story
5. to practise creating novel stories from given ideas or from the child's own imagination that draws on the structure of stories taught in this Section

LP 3 Non-literal language
LP 3.1 Understanding homophones

1. to help the child understand that homophones are words with more than one meaning but which sound the same
2. to develop the child's understanding that homophones can be used to tell jokes
3. to help the child understand that the meaning of homophones in stories and texts is related to the context provided

LP 3.2 Understanding literal and non-literal meanings

1. to help the child understand that idioms are expressions that can be interpreted as a whole; and to demonstrate how to use requests for clarification in understanding idiomatic speech
2. to consolidate idiom understanding and practise using chosen or personalised idioms

LP 3.3 Understanding non-literal meanings in context

1. to engage the child in recognising and understanding the social contexts where idioms are used
2. to help the child understand when idioms and idiomatic language have been used in situations recently or regularly experienced and to use requests for clarification in understanding idiomatic speech

LP 4 Discourse comprehension
LP 4.1 Improving memory and listening

1. to encourage the child to use taught working memory strategies to listen to longer and more complex verbal information

LP 4.2 Understanding verbal inferences

1. to help the child understand 'why–because' reasoning in pictures and answer why questions using the word because
2. to develop the child's understanding of inferences from simple verbal information when no visual context is provided
3. to help the child learn how to identify words in text that he doesn't know and how to use the meaning of the sentence to work out the meaning of the unknown word
4. to help the child develop skills in listening actively to stories and making inferences from spoken texts

LP 4.3 Understanding stories

1. to help the child understand that stories can be broken down into different elements; and be able to answer questions on key factors such as characters, main events, purpose, motivations, and resolutions
2. to develop the child's ability to integrate information from oral stories and make predictions for how the story can end
3. to help the child use the strategy of looking back at the picture or text of a story to check information and to engage actively in building representations of stories
4. to help the child understand how to build mental representations of stories to assist comprehension and to develop awareness of how this helps comprehension

LP 5 Enhanced comprehension monitoring

LP 5.1 Text level comprehension monitoring

1. to assist the child to identify reasons for comprehension challenges in sentences and practise positive strategies for self-help

LP 5.2 Task based comprehension monitoring

1. to develop the child's ability to ask for clarification in tasks which require listening to instructions

SUSI INTERVENTION CONTENT TABLES AND ACTIVITIES

Social Understanding and Social Interpretation (SUSI) content table

Social Understanding and Social Interpretation (SUSI)				
Sections	*Objectives*			
SUSI 1 **Understanding social context cues in interactions**	SUSI 1.1 Understanding non-verbal cues in context	SUSI 1.2 Strategies for problem-solving in simple social communication contexts		
SUSI 2 **Understanding emotion cues in interactions**	SUSI 2.1 Building emotion vocabulary	SUSI 2.2 Enhanced emotion vocabulary	SUSI 2.3 Understanding complex feelings	
SUSI 3 **Understanding and practising flexibility**	SUSI 3.1 Understanding routines	SUSI 3.2 Understanding unplanned change	SUSI 3.3 Making changes in personal routines	
SUSI 4 **Understanding thoughts and intentions of others**	SUSI 4.1 Signalling feelings and intentions (non-verbal)	SUSI 4.2 Predicting thoughts and intentions	SUSI 4.3 Understanding mismatch of language and thoughts	SUSI 4.4 Understanding complex intentions
SUSI 5 **Understanding friendship**	SUSI 5.1 Understanding interests in friendship	SUSI 5.2 Understanding the impact of preferred interests	SUSI 5.3 Understanding friendship skills	

DOI: 10.4324/9781032706641-4

SUSI 1 Intervention content table

SCIP Phase 2	SUSI 1 Intervention content table

SUSI 1 Understanding social context cues in interactions

SUSI 1 Information

SUSI 1.1 Understanding non-verbal cues in context

1 Understanding eye gaze and pointing as intention

2 Understanding social context cues

3 Understanding social context cues (personalised)

SUSI 1.2 Strategies for problem-solving in simple social communication contexts

1 Identifying simple problems in social situations plus Resource

2 Identifying simple problems in social situations (personalised)

SCIP Phase 2: SUSI 1

Information

SUSI 1 Understanding social context cues in interactions

The purpose of this Section is to help your child understand the meaning of non-verbal signals and cues in the social context. Being able to read the social meaning of non-verbal signals means that your child can work out the thoughts, feelings, and intentions of others. This is an important skill for social interaction. Understanding social cues in interactions supports the development of shared knowledge between people and is an important skill for the development of reciprocal relationships and friendships. An understanding of the social cues enables your child to join in with other children.

Work in this Section develops your child's understanding and use of eye gaze and facial expressions to signal thoughts and intentions. The ability to make predictions about probable future events, emotions, and thoughts based on the available social cues will be taught.

Teaching will start by using pictures of one person in a situation that is not problematic in any way. The prediction will not involve problem-solving. Once your child can make simple predictions by reading the social cues, activities are introduced to teach your child how to recognise simple problems in social contexts and to generate solutions to repair the situation or make changes. Gradually as your child works, pictures with two or more people, some with more subtle cues and some with simple problems, will be used. This Section introduces your child to the idea that mild upsets are easily fixed and teaches useful moderating phrases such as, 'never mind', 'oh dear', 'let's try ... instead'.

The order of teaching will be:

- ❖ one person no problem
- ❖ one person with a problem to solve
- ❖ two people no problem
- ❖ two people with a problem to solve
- ❖ more than two people no problem
- ❖ more than two people with a problem to solve

To help with generalisation, recent actual experiences in your child's life will be used to enable your child to transfer these skills to understanding the non-verbal cues in his/her own social interactions.

How you can help

Teaching in this Section can be tailored to meet your child's needs. Please provide information from your child's recent actual experiences when he has found reading social cues challenging. The teaching can incorporate working on understanding these social cues and use similar social contexts to support him to generalise the skills to everyday life. When your child has developed some understanding of these skills, you can play simple games that require understanding and sending non-verbal messages. Your practitioner will advise on how to do this.

SCIP Phase 2: SUSI 1

SUSI 1.1 Understanding non-verbal cues in context

Activity 1: Understanding eye gaze and pointing as intention

Purpose and target

To help the child understand how eye gaze can signal an intention. The child will be able to use eye gaze as a non-verbal means of communicating basic social intentions to other people.

Materials

Pictures of people in different locations using eye gaze to signal an intention. Select useful pictures from *Think It–Say It* by Luanne Martin, Schubi Tell Me About It and Sentimage, Black Sheep Press 3- and 4-step sequences. Start by using pictures showing one person in a situation that is not problematic.

Pictures of people pointing at something or someone.

Blank paper and pens.

Procedure

Select one picture and draw the child's attention to the character's eye gaze. Say, "We are going to work out what this person is thinking by looking at their eyes".

Say, "Look at this boy; he is looking at the biscuit tin. That means he is thinking about the biscuits. What could he be thinking? That's right, he probably wants a biscuit. Let's draw that".

Draw a line between the boy's eyes and the biscuit tin.

Draw a thinking bubble and add the words, 'I want a biscuit'.

Draw a picture of the boy eating a biscuit and put these together with the stimulus picture.

Explain that we know what he is thinking by working out what he is looking at.

Select another picture and repeat the process of making the line between eye gaze and thoughts clear.

Gradually ask the child to make suggestions as to the characters' intentions.

Repeat with pictures of people pointing at something. Write 'I want the X', in the thought bubble for this character.

If useful, obscure the object at the end of the point or eye gaze and ask the child to work out what it could be from other cues in the picture.

SCIP Phase 2: SUSI 1

SUSI 1.1 Understanding non-verbal cues in context

Activity 2: Understanding social context cues

Purpose and target

To help the child understand how to recognise cues in the social context in order to read social meanings.

Materials

Pictures selected from *Think It–Say It* by Luanne Martin or similar scenarios showing at least one person acting in a location.

A checklist of wh- questions to guide the search for social cues (who, where, what is happening? etc.).

Procedure

Lay out one scene and describe how to look for clues in the picture that help explain what is going to happen next. Explain that this is called 'working out what will probably happen'.

Talk about all aspects of the picture and refer to the questions as you explain, e.g., "I know who is in the picture because I can see the man. I know where he is because I can see the cooker and the cupboards, that means he is in the kitchen. I know that he is making toast because he is looking at the toaster. I know that he is not happy because his face looks sad".

Talk about all of these clues as being linked together. These clues go together to help us work out what is happening. He is looking sad and looking at the toaster. Something has happened with his toaster or his toast to make him feel sad. I wonder why he is sad?

Explain that the toaster might be broken. Then show that there is another clue, smoke coming out of it. Ask, "When does smoke come out of the toaster? When the toast is burning, that's right. Oh no! The man has burnt his toast. That would make him sad. I think he is sad because he has burnt his toast. His breakfast is ruined".

Explain how the clues go together to help you to work out what will happen next, what people are thinking, and how the people feel.

Discuss what the man could do to change things.

Draw the predicted events on the white card and as you add details, repeat how you know this will probably happen.

Reinforce the idea of needing more than one clue as you work through the other pictures.

Emphasise that, even when you can't see what will happen, you can "work it out" by "looking for clues". Discourage the use of word guessing so that the child becomes aware of the process of working out.

SCIP Phase 2: SUSI 1

SUSI 1.1 Understanding non-verbal cues in context

Activity 3: Understanding social context cues (personalised)

Purpose and target

To support the child to be able identify and describe expected future events, emotions, and thoughts for recent personal experiences.

Materials

Plain paper and pens to draw simple pictures to represent the child's recent social experiences in school and at home. These should not be challenging situations. For example, draw a classroom with heavy rain visible outside, a new student in class, playing at home, getting ready for an outing.

Speech bubble and arrow-shaped sticky notes.

Procedure

Repeat the procedure for SUSI 1.1 Activity 2.

Say, "Last time we were looking for clues to work out what might happen next. Let's see if you can work out what is going to happen in these stories about your class/family".

Refer to the first scene, "Here is your teacher, and she is looking out of the window. She looks sad. It is raining. I think she is thinking about the rain. I think she is thinking that the children will get wet at playtime. She will say, 'It's inside playtime today'".

Draw children with faces showing different feelings about the rain.

Say, "Look, these children are looking outside as well. Some look happy about the rain and some look sad about it".

Discuss what each might be thinking, e.g., 'no football', 'arts and crafts', and add these to the thinking bubbles.

Draw another figure and say, "This is you; you are looking out at the rain. What are you thinking?".

Ask the child to tell you about what he is looking at, thinking about, will say, etc.

Draw the child's thoughts and words and predicted next actions and discuss.

Explain how the clues help you to work out what will happen next, what people are thinking, and how the people feel.

Draw the predicted events on blank card and, as you add details, repeat how you know this will probably happen.

Record some examples in the child's workbook and gather more examples from parents and teachers if necessary.

SCIP Phase 2: SUSI 1

SUSI 1.2 Strategies for problem-solving in simple social communication contexts

Activity 1: Identifying simple problems in social situations

Purpose and target

To help the child identify that simple problems can be easily fixed and be able to generate possible solutions to given social scenarios.

The child will be taught useful moderating phrases such as, 'never mind', 'oh dear', 'let's try …' to help moderate the emotional response to problems.

Materials

Pictures as described within the Activity 1 Resource.

Procedure

Present one scene and describe the problem to the child.

Highlight the facial expressions of all people in the picture.

Refer back to being able to work out what will probably happen and come up with an ending that is not ideal, asking the child to make predictions as in SUSI 1.1 activities.

Generate several solutions pointing out what can be done and what cannot be fixed.

Discuss how it is usual that such problems happen from time to time.

It is important to highlight that there is more than one solution and that some solutions are better than others.

Introduce the idea of three possible endings, a 'sad ending' where the situation ends badly or gets worse; a 'good ending' finding a solution so that everyone is happy, and an 'OK ending'. An OK ending is one where things are OK for everyone. Introduce set phrases, 'It doesn't matter', 'It's OK', 'Oh well, never mind', etc.

Write or draw all three endings and add speech and thinking bubbles to indicate what is happening. Use key phrases and colour coding to indicate different outcomes e.g., blue for OK, green for good, red for worse. Support the child to be able to weigh up the options.

Start a role-play to demonstrate the sad, OK, and happy endings. Say, "Let's start by making things even worse and making a sad ending. e.g., This boy decides to go home because he isn't in fancy dress. He will miss the party".

Discuss each ending as you act out different choices the child can make.

Record useful words to use and how to ask for help in the child's book.

Use phrases like, 'Think it through', 'Oh, dear, what can we do?', 'We'll just have to do something else instead', 'Everyone makes mistakes, it's OK', 'Never mind, nothing we can do', etc. and talk about how to feel OK about a problem we can't fix.

Repeat with a few scenarios.

As the child becomes confident with this activity, begin to discuss how to prevent something happening again, using 'next time' as a starter phrase.

SCIP Phase 2: SUSI 1

Resource

SUSI 1.2 Strategies for problem-solving in simple social communication contexts

Activity 1 Resource: Identifying simple problems in social situations

This activity is designed to enable the child to recognise simple problems in social contexts and begin to consider solutions.

Draw these scenarios on a sheet of paper leaving at least half the page blank:

- ❖ invited to a swimming party but you forget your towel
- ❖ only one not in fancy dress at a party
- ❖ forgetting your friend's birthday card when you get to his party
- ❖ not getting to unwrap a present in pass the parcel
- ❖ bringing the same present as your friend
- ❖ the only person in uniform on a non-uniform day
- ❖ give the wrong answer in class
- ❖ forget your swimming or sports kit
- ❖ you have not done your homework
- ❖ you do not win a race on Sports day

Leave space above each person's head to add thinking bubbles. Start talking about the first picture and explain that sometimes things don't go to plan. There's a bit of an upset and we need to think about the best thing we can do. It might not be perfect, but it will be OK.

Example: Swimming party

Situation – There is a birthday party at the local swimming baths.

Problem – Child forgets swimming towel.

Discuss – Why this is a problem – because I can't go in the water, I won't be able to get dried after the party.

Discuss some options: Going home and missing all the fun, or staying and enjoy the party in another way, or asking mum to go back home to get a towel or asking a friend if they have a spare towel.

Consider and record how the child can join in and make a contribution to the day without a towel, e.g., being a cheerleader/collecting floats or armbands/giving out balls or water toys.

SCIP Phase 2: SUSI 1

SUSI 1.2 Strategies for problem-solving in simple social communication contexts

Activity 2: Identifying simple problems in social situations (personalised)

Purpose and target

To introduce the child to the idea that he can resolve simple problems in his own experiences.

Materials

Blank paper and pens.
List of recent minor upsets from the child's ISCP.

Procedure

Use only a minor upset and one that was resolved at the time so that there is no lingering upset for the child.

Explain the task: "Last time we talked about the ways in which sometimes things go a bit wrong, and we need to think it through and come up with a good idea to make it OK".

Say, "I know that last week you brought pictures of your new puppy to show your friend Jenna, but she was off school. Jenna was poorly on that day. You were a bit upset. Let's draw that".

Draw the child at school with the pictures of the puppy and draw Jenna at home in bed feeling poorly.

Draw what the child wanted to happen and then ask the child to cross that picture out and say, "That can't happen today because Jenna is poorly".

Now draw what did happen, being a bit upset, and then a good idea from the teacher

Now ask the child to think of some other ways that he could have fixed it.

Discuss a few ideas: Keep the pictures in school, in your book bag, bring them back tomorrow, etc. Talk about how the child was able to come up with good ideas to fix it and talk about how next time that happens he can just say, "OK, I can show her tomorrow".

SCIP Phase 2 | **SUSI 2 Intervention content table**

SUSI 2 Understanding emotion cues in interactions

SUSI 2 Information

SUSI 2.1 Building emotion vocabulary

1 Understanding feelings in social contexts

2 Understanding vocabulary for intensity of feelings

3 Understanding individual emotion reactions to events

4 Understanding matching of reactions to events

SUSI 2.2 Enhanced emotion vocabulary

1 Abstract descriptions of emotions plus Resource

2 Using idioms for emotions

SUSI 2.3 Understanding complex feelings

1 Understanding feelings in complex social contexts plus Resource

2 Solving problems in complex social contexts

3 Solving problems in complex social contexts (personalised)

SCIP Phase 2: SUSI 2

Information

SUSI 2 Understanding emotion cues in interations

The purpose of this Section is to help your child understand words for emotions and how they are linked to events and other people. Being able to make predictions about probable emotions based on the available social cues is an important social ability that enhances the quality of social interactions. This Section creates a Book of Feelings that can be updated and used to discuss and resolve challenges.

Work in this Section develops your child's understanding of the different emotions that arise in different circumstances and explains why different people may have different feelings about the same events. Visual representations for emotions will be used to help your child understand and discuss different emotions and the reasons they arise.

Your child will be taught specific vocabulary for emotions and will learn about differences in intensity of emotion using a visual representation called an emotions ladder. Each emotion ladder shows a range of words for each feeling arranged in order to show stronger emotions at the top and decreasing in intensity to the bottom of the ladder where the feeling is shown as 'OK'. Images and idioms for emotions are included. Learning about the 'size' of the emotion is supported by using different sized symbols for each emotion.

Work in this Section can be collated in a Book of Feelings with a different section for each feeling. Within each section the main concepts of linking feelings with events, language and thoughts, and strength of feeling will be shown. The book will also provide your child with a variety of ways to express and record feelings and events as they arise. Recent actual experiences in your child's life will be used to enable your child to understand the emotion cues in his/her own social interactions and to identify any mismatches between emotion and context.

How you can help

Teaching in this Section can be tailored to meet your child's needs. Please provide information from your child's recent actual experiences on how they react emotionally to different situations, including details of over-reactions to events. Teaching can incorporate working on understanding these emotions and use similar social contexts to support generalisation of these skills to everyday life. Please provide information on the emotion words that your child will be familiar with and any idioms, images, or objects that have meaning for your child. Share successful calming strategies and engage in discussion about developing new calming strategies with the practitioner. Discuss the Book of Feelings with your child and add events as they arise to enrich this book as a meaningful resource. Follow the child's lead in using colour and images to record and represent different emotions.

SCIP Phase 2: SUSI 2

SUSI 2.1 Building emotion vocabulary

Activity 1: Understanding feelings in social contexts

Purpose and target

The child will be able to identify expected emotions for simple social contexts and describe a social situation that would give rise to a specified emotion.

Materials

Photos of happy, sad, angry, and scared faces, e.g., Emotions Fun Deck or similar.

Pictures of events for each emotion e.g., Black Sheep Press Practical Pragmatics.

Speech bubble and thought bubble sticky notes.

Notebook divided into sections for each emotion to be targeted in Phase 2.

This activity forms the first part of making a Book of Feelings for use throughout Phase 2. This activity should be repeated until all emotions being targeted in Phase 2 have been covered and added to the Book of Feelings.

Procedure

Explain that the child needs to listen and work out which feeling you are talking about.

Lay out up to four emotion photo cards and name each one as you place it down.

Describe an event in terms of what is happening and ask the child to match to the feeling.

Show the child the scene and discuss the event, facial expressions of characters, and the feeling words that best match the event. Support as necessary by modelling or giving choices or words.

Begin to introduce different words for intensity in preparation for Activity 2.

Repeat for all four emotions with several examples from the events pictures.

Role-reversal

Give the child a set of event cards and ask the child to select one and describe it for you to match to the emotion.

Repeat until the child has been able to describe events for all the targeted feelings.

Support the child to provide descriptions of events and reasons for feelings.

Meta-challenge

Ask the child to repeat this again but now insert a meta-challenge into the game by providing
wrong answers to the child's descriptions and observe his response to this. Support him
to correct you and to explain why your answer didn't match. Make this fun.

When the child has shown an awareness of events and emotions begin to discuss solutions
for emotions such as anger, sadness, and fear in preparation for SUSI 2.3 Activity 2

Create the child's Book of Feelings

Divide the notebook into sections, one for each emotion. For each emotion section, write
the name of the feeling and draw a large face to represent this feeling on the first
page. On the following pages add some events just discussed that provoke this feeling.
Leave enough pages within each section to keep adding new learning and outputs from
activities as you progress through SUSI 2.

SCIP Phase 2: SUSI 2

SUSI 2.1 Building emotion vocabularry

Activity 2: Understanding vocabulary for intensity of feelings

Purpose and target

To help the child understand that feelings differ in intensity and to learn words to express these differing intensities using a visual representation for support.

Materials

Blank outline of emotion ladders for happy, sad, angry, scared with up to five rungs for five graded emotion words (and other targeted emotions as needed).

Symbols, photos, or drawings to represent emotions.

At least three pictures of events for each feeling graded for intensity, e.g., from Schubi Sentimage or Black Sheep Press Practical Pragmatics.

Age-appropriate thesaurus or lists of differing intensity emotion words for each emotion.

Child's Book of Feelings from Activity 1: This activity forms one part of making a Book of Feelings for use throughout Phase 2. This activity should be repeated until all emotions being targeted in Phase 2 have been covered and added to the Book of Feelings.

Procedure

Start with happy feelings. Select pictures of events that will provoke a differing intensity of happiness, e.g., you feel *pleased* to have an ice-cream, going to a birthday party makes you *happy*, having your own birthday party makes you feel *excited* and *joyful*.

Write the events and emotion words in order on the child's emotions ladder.

Draw large or small feeling faces to represent the change in intensity beside the event.

Write the words in smaller or larger size, or darker or lighter colours, to illustrate the intensity of the feelings.

Explain that the position of each emotion on the ladder has meaning, strong feelings are at the top, smaller feelings are close to the bottom and close to 'feeling OK'.

Together with the child, name a range of words for this feeling and discuss suitable events that would provoke each emotion.

Use the thesaurus if appropriate for the child.

Aim to come up with a minimum of three words that can be graded for each feeling, but extend in line with the child's ability and needs.

Repeat with event pictures and graded emotion vocabulary for all feelings targeted.

Encourage the child to contribute ideas for how he can express intensity of feelings in a visual way.

Personalisation

Use words that are meaningful for the child collected from the child's ISCP or from recent parent or teacher report.

Encourage logical positioning of feelings on the ladders, e.g., worried below scared, but adjust depending on the child's views, e.g., frustrated above or below angry, etc.

Discuss events that may lead to these feelings in general terms and note if the child volunteers information on events they have experienced and add these to the ISCP.

SCIP Phase 2: SUSI 2

SUSI 2.1 Building emotion vocabulary

Activity 3: Understanding individual emotional reactions to events

Purpose and target

To help the child understand that feelings differ in intensity depending on the event and what it means to each person.

Materials

Pictures of events for each feeling from Schubi Sentimage or Black Sheep Press.
Age-appropriate thesaurus.
Plain paper and pens to draw character's emotional responses to the events.
Emotion ladders created in Activity 2.
Child's Book of Feelings from Activity 1: This activity forms one part of making a Book of Feelings for use throughout Phase 2. This activity should be repeated until all emotions being targeted in Phase 2 have been covered and added to the Book of Feelings.

Procedure

Start by looking at the emotion ladders created in Activity 2 and the pictures of events that indicate the differing intensity of feeling.

Present a new event and draw two or three characters on a single A4 page.

Explain that although the event makes all characters feel e.g., scared, that they each react to the situation differently. Include a character who will feel OK. For example, most of the children are scared of the spider. Tom is *terrified* of spiders and will run away and scream for help. Jane is *scared* and will leave the room to avoid being near it. Marcia is only a little *worried* and will carry on playing and try not to think about it. Jack likes spiders so he will feel *OK*. Illustrate this using a thinking bubble for each character.

Refer to the emotions ladder and show where each child's feeling is located. Draw a line from the child's face to the emotion word for their experience and add the emotion word to their thinking bubble either as a single word or as a sentence.

Repeat using another event for the same emotion and draw this out as an example in the child's Book of Feelings. For example, Tom is not scared of the barking dogs because he has had a dog as a pet and knows that dogs bark when they hear people coming to their house. He knows that most dogs don't bite people. He feels *OK*. Marcia has never owned a dog and is sure the dog will bite; she is *frightened* and will hide behind her Mum. Jane was chased by a dog in the park and is now *terrified* of all dogs; she will run away screaming.

Using the same characters, show that children react differently to different events within the same emotion. For example, show that someone who was terrified of dogs is not scared at all on the rollercoaster, or terrified on the rollercoaster and OK on the tree-line walk, etc.

Explain that not all scared feelings are the same size and not everyone is scared of the same things.

Engage the child in coming up with events that would provoke differing strengths of reactions and in giving reasons why the strength of feeling might be different for each character.

Repeat using at least three events for each emotion and repeat this activity to cover all targeted emotions in Phase 2.

SCIP Phase 2: SUSI 2

SUSI 2.1 Building emotion vocabulary

Activity 4: Understanding matching of reactions to events

Purpose and target

To help the child understand the idea of over-reactions to events and that emotional reactions usually match the event.

Materials

Pictures of events as for Activity 3.

Two or three characters, e.g., laminated figures of different boys and girls.

Child's Book of Feelings from Activity 1: This activity forms one part of making a Book of Feelings for use throughout Phase 2. This activity should be repeated until all emotions being targeted in Phase 2 have been covered and added to the Book of Feelings.

Procedure

Start by looking at the emotions ladder created in Activity 2 and the pictures of events that match the differing intensities of feeling.

Present an event that has been agreed as producing a moderate reaction and one new character.

Explain that the event makes everyone feel e.g., scared, but this boy over-reacts. Say, "Over-reacts means that he is more scared than he needs to be. The feeling is too big for what is happening. It's only a small spider on the bath; there's no need to scream and cry and shout for Mummy".

Draw a picture of the event and two different facial expressions, a scared face and a terrified face.

Explain that being scared is the right feeling, but that terrified is too strong/too big.

Exaggerate the visual detail, e.g., a very small spider in a bath with a large, very scared face. Say, these don't match. The feeling is too big.

Add language to moderate the reaction and come up with solutions, e.g., "It's OK; it won't bite my head off", "It can't catch me", "I can leave it to get on with making a web and tell Mum it's there", "No worries", etc.

Emphasise the vocabulary of reaction that the feeling is right, the size of the feeling needs to be smaller. Explain that this is the "right feeling, but the wrong size". This validates the feeling and asks for an evaluation of the reaction size.

On a fresh emotions ladder mark the reaction at a point higher than the expected reaction.

Add an arrow pointing downwards from the reaction to the expected reaction.

Use a gesture to represent dropping the feeling size down the ladder as you discuss.

In discussion, explain that this is usually because the problem is easily fixed.

Repeat with other examples for fear before moving on to over-reactions for other emotions, e.g., too excited, overly angry, and overly upset, and repeat the process adding at least one example to the child's Book of Feelings as you work.

SCIP Phase 2: SUSI 2

SUSI 2.2 Enhanced emotion vocabulary

Activity 1: Abstract descriptions of emotions

Purpose and target

To help the child understand that emotions can be conceptualised and described in abstract terms and through images.

Materials

Photos of all emotions worked on in SUSI 2.

Activity 1 Resource for examples of words, images, and objects that can be used as abstract representations.

Information from the child's ISCP to personalise this activity.

Emotions ladders from Activity 2.

Child's Book of Feelings from Activity 1: This activity forms one part of making a Book of Feelings for use throughout Phase 2. This activity should be repeated until all emotions being targeted in Phase 2 have been covered and added to the Book of Feelings.

Procedure

Work through one emotion at a time and explain that today we are going to use our imagination to think of images and other words that can signal an emotion.

Start with happy and provide a range of images that can be used to signify feeling happy, e.g., smiling face, sunshine, blue sky, beach scene or sandcastle, present wrapped in a big bow, cuddling a pet, etc.

Explain that we know that these images mean happy because most people would feel happy when they think of these things.

Personalisation

Use information from the child's ISCP in consultation with the child, e.g., "I know that you play table tennis every week. We can use a drawing of table tennis to show how happy you feel when you play". Talk this through in depth to determine the intensity of feeling associated with these activities and link the word, e.g., I feel happy/delighted when I play table tennis.

Make links to the emotions ladder throughout and add any illustrations that are meaningful for the child to the emotions ladders.

Repeat the process for all targeted emotions in Phase 2 and add at least one example to the child's Book of Feelings as you work.

SCIP Phase 2: SUSI 2

Resource

SUSI 2.2 Enhanced emotion vocabulary

Activity 1 Resource: Abstract descriptions of emotions

This activity is designed to enable the child to understand and use abstract images and words for feelings.

Create a set of words and images appropriate to the needs of the child from the suggestions below.

Happy

Joyful	Pleased	Contented	Light as a feather	Smiling
Feather	Sunshine	Sandcastle	Bike or favourite toy	Sweets or chocolate treat

Sad

Miserable	Tearful	Crying	Down in the dumps
Raincloud	Puddles	Broken toy	No-one to play with

Angry

Cross	Mad	Frustrated	Shouting
Thunderbolt	Hammer	Drum kit	Megaphone

Afraid

Worried	Frightened	Anxious	Shaking
Wobbly jelly	Shaking legs Spider	Tall ladder	

Excited

Energetic	Enthusiastic	Bouncy	Looking forward to something
Firework	Rollercoaster	Gift	Jumping up and down

Relaxed

Chilled out	Comfortable	Casual	Carefree
Big armchair	Favourite pet	Lying on the floor	Sunny garden

SCIP Phase 2: SUSI 2

SUSI 2.2 Enhanced emotion vocabulary

Activity 2: Using idioms for emotions

Purpose and target

To help the child use idioms to describe emotions as a way of conceptualising and describing emotions in abstract terms.

Materials

Pictures of idioms for emotions selected from *120 Idioms at Your Fingertips*, or similar resource.

List of idioms for emotions from Activity 2 Resource.

Emotions ladders from Activity 2.

Child's Book of Feelings from Activity 1: This activity forms one part of making a Book of Feelings for use throughout Phase 2. This activity should be repeated until all emotions being targeted in Phase 2 have been covered and added to the Book of Feelings.

Procedure

Explain that sometimes people use sayings or expressions to describe how they are feeling.

Say, "Someone might say 'I am over the moon' when she is very happy, or she might say 'I am down in the dumps' when she means she is feeling sad".

Show the pictures and stick these into the child's Book of Feelings under happy and sad respectively.

Present another idiom and explain the non-literal meaning and the related emotion.

Ask if the child knows any idioms for feelings and draw these into the child's Book of Feelings in the matching emotion section.

Ask parents and teachers for examples that the child might be familiar with.

Make links to the emotions ladders throughout.

Ask parents and teachers to deliberately use idioms to talk about feelings in context and to talk about these with the child, e.g., "I bet you feel on top of the world after winning the school cup".

SCIP Phase 2: SUSI 2

Resource

SUSI 2.2 Enhanced emotion vocabulary

Activity 2 Resource: Using idioms for emotions

Happy

- ❖ over the moon/tickled pink
- ❖ full of beans/feeling like the bee's knees
- ❖ on top of the world/walking on air
- ❖ grinning like a cat that got the cream

Sad

- ❖ down in the dumps/have a long face
- ❖ feeling blue/feeling low
- ❖ under a cloud/having a grey day
- ❖ cry your eyes out/heartbroken

Angry

- ❖ you are in my bad books/bite your head off
- ❖ have a bee in your bonnet/lose your head
- ❖ get out of the wrong side of the bed
- ❖ she hit the roof/blow your top
- ❖ his bark is worse than his bite

Scared

- ❖ jump out of my skin/shaking in my shoes/knees knocking
- ❖ keep your fingers crossed/cross that bridge when you get to it
- ❖ get it off your chest/have butterflies in your tummy
- ❖ it is not the end of the world

Relaxed and calm

- ❖ cool as a cucumber
- ❖ chilling out/laid back

❖ water off a duck's back

Over-reaction

❖ don't make a mountain out of a molehill
❖ a storm in a teacup
❖ to get worked up about something

Tired

❖ he's been burning the candle at both ends
❖ ready to drop/out like a light/sleep like a log

SCIP Phase 2: SUSI 2

SUSI 2.3 Understanding complex feelings

Activity 1: Understanding feelings in complex social contexts

Purpose and target

To help the child identify expected emotions for a range of social contexts. To enable the child to describe a social situation that would give rise to a specified emotion.

Materials

Photos of disappointed, embarrassed, worried, surprised, frustrated, and confused faces, e.g., Emotions Fun Deck.

Pictures of events for each of these emotions, e.g., Winslow Colorcards Emotions.

Speech bubble and thought bubble sticky notes.

Activity 1 Resource.

Emotions ladders from Activity 2.

Child's Book of Feelings from Activity 1: This activity forms one part of making a Book of Feelings for use throughout Phase 2. This activity should be repeated until all emotions being targeted in Phase 2 have been covered and added to the Book of Feelings.

Procedure

Explain that the child needs to listen and work out which feeling you are talking about.

Lay out up to four emotion photo cards and name each one as you place it down.

Describe an event from the Activity Resource that matches one of the emotions.

Ask the child to point to the emotion you are talking about.

If you have a suitable context photo, show the child the scene and discuss the event, facial expressions of characters, and the feeling words that best match the event.

Discuss the situation and why the emotion matches the situation.

Repeat for all emotions with several examples from the events pictures.

When the child has shown an awareness of events and emotions, begin to discuss solutions for each of the emotions targeted.

Role-reversal

Give the child the emotion cards and ask him to describe "what might happen to make someone feel this way" for you to work out the emotion.

Repeat until the child has been able to describe events for all the targeted feelings.

Support the child to provide descriptions of events and reasons for feelings as needed.

Meta-challenge

Ask the child to repeat this again but now provide a meta-challenge by introducing mismatched answers to the child's descriptions and observe his response to this. Support him to identify why your answer was mismatched. Make this fun.

Personalisation

Depending on the child's needs create a section in the Book of Feelings for 'tricky feelings' and add at least one example of each emotion covered as you work. For some children a more expansive section on e.g., frustrated or worried might be needed.

SCIP Phase 2: SUSI 2

Resource

SUSI 2.3 Understanding complex feelings

Activity 1 Resource: Understanding feelings in complex social contexts

This activity is designed to develop understanding of feelings in complex contexts.

Scripts for complex emotional scenarios:

Disappointed

❖ someone wants a new bike for his birthday, but he gets a scooter
❖ someone wants his friend to sleep at his house, but he has to go home
❖ someone wants to have pizza for lunch, but it's all gone when he gets to the counter
❖ someone wanted to win the competition, but he came third

Embarrassed

❖ someone has lost his friend's ball
❖ someone has burped loudly in class by mistake
❖ someone got the answer wrong when the teacher asked him a question
❖ someone is wearing her jumper inside out

Worried

❖ someone thinks his best friend doesn't want to play with him
❖ someone is waiting for his dad to pick him up after school, but he is late
❖ someone is late for school
❖ someone can't find his mum in the supermarket

Surprised

❖ someone thought he was getting a book from his auntie, but it's a ticket to see his favourite football team play
❖ someone won a prize in the school raffle
❖ someone was picked to be captain of the football team
❖ someone has planned a surprise birthday party

Frustrated

- ❖ someone is waiting at the traffic lights for a long time
- ❖ someone didn't have enough time to finish her work before playtime
- ❖ someone can't score a goal
- ❖ someone is not tall enough for the ride at the funfair

Confused

- ❖ someone doesn't know what to do in class
- ❖ someone is playing a new game that has lots of rules
- ❖ someone is making a model aeroplane and it's very complicated
- ❖ someone doesn't know where the paints are stored in class

SCIP Phase 2: SUSI 2

SUSI 2.3 Understanding complex feelings

Activity 2: Solving problems in complex social contexts

Purpose and target

To facilitate the child's understanding of matching emotions for complex social situations; to help the child describe expected emotions, thoughts, and words for complex social contexts.

Materials

Photos of emotions: Disappointed, embarrassed, worried, surprised, frustrated, and confused faces, e.g., Emotions Fun Deck.

Pictures of social contexts with complex emotions such as worry, disappointment, surprise, frustration, confusion, or embarrassment, selected from Schubi Sentimage, Tell Me About It or Papa Moll sequence sets; Winslow ColorCards: Skills for Daily Living: Social Behaviour.

Speech bubble and thought bubble sticky notes.

Activity 1 Resource.

Child's Book of Feelings from Activity 1: This activity forms one part of making a Book of Feelings for use throughout Phase 2. This activity should be repeated until all emotions being targeted in Phase 2 have been covered and added to the Book of Feelings.

Procedure

Lay out one social context picture depicting one or more of the emotions listed and describe the picture in detail to explain the events, feelings, predicted thoughts, and intentions. Explain visual inferences in detail and engage the child to describe and predict as much as he can.

Select the matching emotion photo and show that this feeling matches the events in the picture.

Discuss sufficiently to ensure that the child has understood.

Once you have identified the problem and upset, start to focus on working towards solutions using all the emotion vocabulary and ideas that have been taught up to now, e.g., use visuals, idioms and preferred vocabulary, refer to reactions and over-reactions, and repeat 'right feeling, wrong size'. Use set phrases e.g., 'It doesn't matter', 'It's OK', 'Oh well, never mind'.

Ask "What would make it feel better?", "What could he do to help?".

Discuss and write down at least two solutions for each situation.

Record a summary or sketch of the scenario and the solutions in the child's Book of Feelings under the matched emotion/section of the book.

Repeat with at least two pictures for each emotion and until the child can identify the emotion, the problem, and suggest a few solutions for each feeling being targeted.

As the child becomes confident with this activity, begin to discuss how to prevent something happening again, using 'next time' as a starter phrase.

If the child volunteers information relating to their experience of these emotions add to the ISCP and use in Activity 3.

SCIP Phase 2: SUSI 2

SUSI 2.3 Understanding complex feelings

Activity 3: Solving problems in complex social contexts (personalised)

Purpose and target

To facilitate the child's understanding of his own emotional reactions in complex social situations; to help the child to describe his own and others' perspectives and suggest solutions for emotional reactions.

Materials

Ideas of recent upsets and emotional reactions to events and misunderstandings of events from the child's ISCP or from recent parent/teacher report.

Child's Book of Feelings.

Procedure

This activity needs to be sensitively managed, preferably when a strong alliance has been established and the child is robust enough to cope with direct feedback.

Explain the task: "Last time we talked about the ways in which people sometimes feel upset, embarrassed, worried, and disappointed, and we came up with ideas to help them feel better. Today we are going to talk about things that happen to you and help you come up with ideas to feel better".

Draw a scenario based on the child's recent experience. For example, "I know that last week when Steven came to your house to play, you got upset when he played with your cars. Here's a picture of you and Steven playing".

Draw each picture and talk the child through the event slowly and carefully, talking about the feeling, does it match the event, yes or no, and explain why. For example, "When we invite our friends to play that means they can play with our toys. Playing with our friends makes us feel happy. Part of playing together is sharing the toys. Being upset doesn't match. Oh dear. What can we say, do, or think to fix that?".

Add thinking and speech bubbles to add detail as you expand the sequence of events.

Provide solutions, "I want to play with Steven, so he can play with my cars. We can both play with the cars, we can take turns". "I can say, 'OK your turn', I feel OK about sharing my toys".

Or, for example, "Last week, I know that badminton club was full, and you didn't get a place. You were disappointed. That's the right feeling. You cried and shouted and threw a book on the floor. That's a big reaction. That was too big for this disappointment. Let's think what you could do instead. It's OK to be disappointed. Let's draw that. This is you, and you are waiting to play badminton. There is a long queue, and you are at the back. When you get to the front the teacher says, 'No more space today, sorry'. You are upset. Let's stop and think what we can do. You can say, 'I really wanted to play', 'Can I play next time?' etc.".

Make links to the emotions ladder throughout and add this as an example to the Book of Feelings under that emotion.

Repeat with a range of situations that have occurred recently and if the child is feeling overwhelmed return to Activity 2 to work on general examples, not personalised examples.

If the child shows some reflective ability and can tolerate working on a personal example, consider how this work can be used to support a Phase 3 target.

| **SCIP Phase 2** | **SUSI 3 Intervention content table** |

SUSI 3 Understanding and practising flexibility

SUSI 3 Information

SUSI 3.1 Understanding routines

1 Understanding vocabulary for routines plus Resource

2 Understanding routines at school plus Resource

3 Understanding routines at home plus Resource

SUSI 3.2 Understanding unplanned change

1 Understanding and coping with accidents plus Resource

2 Understanding unplanned change plus Resource

3 Winning and losing a game

SUSI 3.3 Making changes in personal routines

1 Understanding the impact of being flexible

2 Understanding the impact of being flexible (personalised)

SCIP Phase 2: SUSI 3
Information

SUSI 3 Understanding and practising flexibility

The purpose of this Section is to help your child understand vocabulary and concepts to describe routines, accidents, and unplanned change, and support him to become more accepting of changes to expectations. Concepts of winning and losing, being lucky and unlucky are covered. The vocabulary taught includes the words 'always', 'never', 'sometimes', 'usually', 'often', 'inflexible', and 'flexible'. Visual representations will be used to help your child understand. Routines and expectations associated with the school day and home life are targeted. This Section teaches the impact of being inflexible where changes to routines are explored to consider 'what might happen?' and develop coping strategies.

As your child gains insight to how changes can be managed, work will include situations similar to those your child finds challenging. This aims to support your child to reflect on his/her own adherence to routines and the impact of being inflexible in his/her own life. Simple changes in routines are proposed to enable your child to learn about coping strategies.

Once your child can understand the vocabulary and concepts associated with routines, activities are introduced to teach your child how to understand and reflect on his/her own routines. In discussion with you, small interruptions to routines will be proposed and support offered to generate solutions to accept the change or to stay calm when change happens unexpectedly. Recent actual experiences in your child's life will be used to enable your child to understand the emotion cues in his/her own social interactions and to resolve upsets in his/her own experiences. Work in this Section is supported by the child's Book of Feelings and emotions ladders created in work in SUSI 2.

Routines can be useful and can help children to learn and remember new events. However, it is also important for children to be able to accept that sometimes things don't go to plan. Children can be supported to develop flexibility and coping strategies for unexpected change. Using stories about other people helps prepare your child for thinking about his/her own routines. Discussing routines and mild upsets in detail and away from the actual event can help your child understand and accept change in real-world situations. Having a set phrase that can be used in the real situation can help your child apply the new strategy.

How you can help

Teaching in this Section can be tailored to meet your child's needs. Please provide information on your child's past and current preferred routines and how he reacts emotionally when change happens, including details of over-reactions to events. Please provide details of routines that could be changed without causing upset. Teaching can incorporate working on understanding these events and can use similar social contexts to support generalisation of these skills to everyday life. Please provide information on what steps are taken to avoid change or to repair an upset. Changes to routines need to be managed sensitively. Make change to one routine at a time, starting with one that has little or no emotional import. Close liaison with the practitioner is recommended to support work on change to routines.

SCIP Phase 2: SUSI 3

SUSI 3.1 Understanding routines

Activity 1: Understanding vocabulary for routines

Purpose and target

To help the child understand vocabulary and concepts to describe routines and expectations associated with routines in order to enable him to understand and manage changes in routines.

Materials

Scenarios and vocabulary from the SUSI 3.1 Activity 1 Resource.
Emotions ladders and child's Book of Feelings from SUSI 2.

Procedure

Discuss a few common school- or home-based routines and use the words 'always', 'never', 'sometimes', and 'usually'. Do not discuss changes to routines.

Discuss the worked example as described in the Activity Resource. Explain that sometimes people like to do exactly the same thing every day. Explain that it makes them feel happy and relaxed. Point to these feelings on the emotions ladder.

Write the words 'always' and 'never' on opposite ends of a line (continuum) and point to these as you talk about the routine adding other phrases and words useful for the child's insight and ability to understand.

Explain each step in the routine so that when you discuss solutions you can refer back to each step and see if it can be changed to make things better.

Now introduce the idea of unplanned and unexpected changes to routines.

Emphasise that sometimes things happen that people did not expect and because they did not expect it, they need time to think to work out how to make things better. Explain that this means that they might not like the change, and it might cause them to feel upset.

Discuss thoughts, feelings, and words for the characters and draw these out on a sheet of paper using speech and thought bubbles.

Work towards solutions and acceptance. Make explicit reference to feeling upset, possible solutions, and to the thoughts, feelings, and words for each person as required.

Include a moderating voice for one of the characters and model set phrases, e.g., 'never mind', 'sometimes things change', 'usually I do this, but today I have to do this instead', 'That's OK, never mind', 'There's nothing we can do', etc.

Review the story and use the words 'inflexible' and 'flexible' to describe the behaviour. Point out that being flexible has advantages, but that we need to take 'thinking time' to work out what to do instead.

Link to thoughts and feeling OK about the change.

Work towards the person staying calm and discuss at least two solutions for this situation.

Discuss at least two more changes to routines and record strategies to cope with each.

Refer to emotion changes on emotions ladders.

Record a summary or sketch of one of the changes to routines and the solutions in the child's Book of Feelings under the matching emotion/section of the book.

If the child volunteers information relating to their experience of changes to routines add to the ISCP and use in SUSI 3.3, and explain that you will work on this in a future session.

SCIP Phase 2: SUSI 3
Resource

SUSI 3.1 Understanding routines

Activity 1 Resource: Understanding vocabulary for routines

This activity is designed to teach vocabulary associated with routines and to understand that steps in a routine can be interrupted. Vocabulary to be taught is: 'routine', 'always', 'never', 'sometimes', 'usually', and 'often'. 'Always' and 'never' are linked to being 'inflexible', and 'sometimes' and 'usually' are linked to being 'flexible'. Write these words on separate cards and use drawings as required. Words can be arranged on a continuum with 'always' and 'never' at each extreme and 'usually' and 'sometimes' in the middle.

Draw these scenarios on a sheet of paper leaving at least half the page blank:

* ❖ a man is waiting for the bus to work. It is late
* ❖ there is a diversion on the way to school
* ❖ the batteries in a game or toy are flat
* ❖ a favourite TV programme is not on
* ❖ a favourite ice cream is not available at the shop

Describe the routine as what usually happens and as what the person prefers.

This man *always* gets the bus to work. He gets on at a stop near his house and pays the driver. It takes 20 minutes to get to his office. He starts work at 9.00 a.m. He *always* gets the bus and *never* drives. *This is his routine*. He likes *to stick to his routine*. This means *he likes getting the bus* and *he doesn't like it when he can't get the bus*.

Describe an upset: The bus is usually on time. Sometimes it is a little bit late. He doesn't mind as long as he gets to work on time. Today the bus is late. The man waits at his stop *as usual*, but it doesn't show up. He *is expecting the bus* to come. He *wants to get the bus to work*. That is his routine, *but today he can't*. It's not coming. He is going to be late.

Discuss thoughts and feelings arising from this situation.

Discuss possible solutions: Use another person at the stop as a moderating voice with suggestions on how to get to work on time: Get a different bus and walk further/share a taxi/ phone his colleagues to explain/walk to a different stop.

Explain using phrases that are already in use or agree suitable phrases with parents/teachers. For example, *I can't do anything about it*, *I have to break my routine*, *I need to be flexible*. Sometimes, *it's OK to* get the next bus and walk a bit further to my office. *Never mind, it'll work out fine. It's not ideal, but it's OK for today.* I need thinking time to work out what to do

Review the story and point out that getting the same bus is a fixed routine, there was an unexpected/unplanned change, and that he needed to be flexible to make things better for himself.

Repeat this scenario, but this time as a flexible routine. The man has a variety of ways to get to work and he can choose. For example, in sunny weather he might walk or cycle. Point out that when the bus doesn't come, he can choose some other way to get there. He can choose a different way to get to work and he does not feel upset.

For older children, use idiomatic language to describe routines and expectations, e.g., regular as clockwork, being off timetable, taking a break from routine, try it and see, etc.

SCIP Phase 2: SUSI 3

SUSI 3.1 Understanding routines

Activity 2: Understanding routines at school

Purpose and target

To help the child understand vocabulary and concepts to describe routines and expectations associated with the school day in order to enable him to understand and manage changes in routines.

Materials

Scenarios and vocabulary from the SUSI 3.1 Activity 2 Resource.
Emotions ladders and child's Book of Feelings from SUSI 2.

Procedure

Refer to the usual routine script in the Activity 2 Resource for ideas on what to say for each scene. Do not use a scenario that the child will recognise as challenging and might cause upset at this stage.

Explain that this work is to understand routines at school and what we like about the routines, explaining that changes to routine sometimes happen. Start talking about the first picture and explain that usually the timetable is the same every week. Explain that this is helpful to have the equipment we need and to know what we need to do. It makes us feel happy and relaxed. Point to these feelings on the emotions ladder.

Now explain that a change has happened to the routine, e.g., a visiting sports coach, so no maths lesson today. Discuss thoughts, feelings, and words for how the teacher and the children feel. Draw these out on a sheet of paper using speech and thought bubbles and adding emotion vocabulary the child knows. Add some children who are pleased because they don't like maths, some who are upset because they don't like sports and some who are relaxed, happy, or excited about the change.

As in Activity 1, emphasise and explain that sometimes things happen that people did not expect, might not like, might make them a bit upset, etc. Work toward solutions in terms of thoughts, feelings, and words as before. Model set phrases, e.g., "Sometimes things change, usually the children do this, but today they have to do this instead". "That's OK, never mind", etc. Refer to being flexible and inflexible and the advantages of being flexible.

Work towards children being able to stay calm and discuss strategies for this.

Discuss at least two more changes to routines and write down strategies to cope with each situation. Refer to emotion changes on the emotions ladders.

Record a summary or sketch of one of the changes to routines and the solutions in the child's Book of Feelings under the matching emotion/section of the book.

Role-reversal

Present a scenario as a routine and ask the child to suggest a break in the routine and then to suggest a solution.

If the child volunteers information relating to their experience of changes to routines add to the ISCP and use in SUSI 3.3 and explain that you will work on this in a future session.

SCIP Phase 2: SUSI 3

Resource

SUSI 3.1 Understanding routines

Activity 2 Resource: Understanding routines at school

This activity is designed to teach vocabulary associated with routines at school and to understand that steps in a routine can be interrupted. Vocabulary to be taught is 'routine', 'always', 'never', 'sometimes', 'usually', and 'often'. Write these words on separate cards and use drawings as required. Words can be arranged on a continuum with 'always' and 'never' at each extreme and 'usually' and 'sometimes' in the middle.

Draw these scenarios on a sheet of paper leaving at least half the page blank:

- ❖ a change in the timetable
- ❖ your usual teacher is ill, so there is a replacement teacher
- ❖ Sports Day is cancelled because of bad weather
- ❖ it is too wet to play outside, indoor playtime instead
- ❖ a visit from the school nurse/speech and language therapist, etc. You miss a lesson
- ❖ you have a dentist appointment and have to leave school early or arrive late
- ❖ rehearsals for the school play

Describe what usually happens and the upset to the routine and solutions as in Activity 1.

For older children, use idiomatic language to describe routines and expectations, e.g., regular as clockwork, being off timetable, taking a break from routine, try it and see, etc.

SCIP Phase 2: SUSI 3

SUSI 3.1 Understanding routines

Activity 3: Understanding routines at home

Purpose and target

To help the child understand vocabulary and concepts to describe routines and expectations associated with the home routine, in order to enable him to understand and manage changes in routines.

Materials

Scenarios and vocabulary from the Activity 3 Resource.
Emotions ladders and child's Book of Feelings from SUSI 2.

Procedure

Refer to the 'usual routine' script in the Resource for ideas on what to say for each scene. Do not use a scenario the child will recognise as challenging and might cause upset at this stage.

Explain that this work is to understand routines at home and what we like about the routines and explain that changes to routine sometimes happen. Start talking about the first picture and explain that usually, e.g., we have cereal for breakfast. Explain that it's nice to have our favourite breakfast every day. It makes us feel happy and relaxed. Point to these feelings on the emotions ladder.

Explain that a change has happened to the routine, e.g., no milk so there can be no cereal today. Discuss thoughts, feelings, and words for how everyone might feel. Draw the scenario on a sheet of paper using speech and thought bubbles. Use emotion vocabulary the child knows. Include one child who is pleased (he prefers toast for breakfast); one who is upset (she prefers cereal and wants it); and one who doesn't mind (she is relaxed and happy about the change).

As in Activity 1, emphasise and explain that sometimes things happen that people did not expect, might not like, might make them feel upset, etc. Work towards solutions in terms of thoughts, feelings, and words as before. Model set phrases, e.g., "Sometimes things change, usually the children do this, but today they have to do this instead", "That's OK, never mind", etc. Refer to being flexible and inflexible and the advantages of being flexible. Sometimes it's OK to be flexible, sometimes we have to be flexible, etc.

Work towards children being able to stay calm and discuss strategies for this.

Discuss at least two more changes to routines and write down strategies to cope with each situation. Refer to emotion changes on the emotions ladders.

Record a summary or sketch of one of the changes to routines and the solutions in the child's Book of Feelings under the matching emotion/section of the book.

Role-reversal

Present a scenario as a routine and ask the child to suggest a break in the routine and then to suggest a solution.

If the child volunteers information relating to their experience of changes to routines add to the ISCP and use in SUSI 3.3 and explain that you will work on this in a future session.

SCIP Phase 2: SUSI 3

Resource

SUSI 3.1 Understanding routines

Activity 3 Resource: Understanding routines at home

This activity is designed to teach vocabulary associated with routines at home and to understand that steps in a routine can be interrupted. Vocabulary to be taught is 'routine', 'always', 'never', 'sometimes', 'usually', and 'often'. Write these words on separate cards and use a drawing if that will help. Words can be arranged on a continuum with 'always' and 'never' at each extreme and 'usually' and 'sometimes' in the middle.

Draw these scenarios on a sheet of paper leaving at least half the page blank:

❖ no milk for cereal in the morning. Let's have toast
❖ late home from Grandma's. No time for a bath before bed
❖ the library is closed, and you can't get any new books today
❖ in a hurry to take your sister to a music lesson. No time for games after school
❖ your brother is ill; he's staying at home. You're going to school
❖ it's non-uniform day at school. Get dressed in your favourite clothes

Describe what usually happens and the upset to the routine and solutions as in Activity 1.

For older children, use idiomatic language to describe routines and expectations, e.g., regular as clockwork, being off timetable, taking a break from routine, try it and see, etc.

SCIP Phase 2: SUSI 3

SUSI 3.2 Understanding unplanned change

Activity 1: Understanding and coping with accidents

Purpose and target

To help the child understand vocabulary and concepts associated with accidents, making mistakes, and associated feelings.

Materials

Scenarios and vocabulary from the SUSI 3.2 Activity 1 Resource.
Emotions ladders and child's Book of Feelings from SUSI 2.

Procedure

Refer to the sample script in the Activity 1 Resource for ideas on what to say for each scene. Using the first scene, explain that accidents are things that happen that we didn't plan or want to happen.

When presenting each scenario, talk about the feelings of the person who caused the accident before talking about the feelings of the person who was hurt or upset by the accident. Show that both people have feelings about what happened.

Draw each event on a sheet of paper using speech and thought bubbles. Use emotion vocabulary the child knows and refer to emotions ladders as you work for both characters.

Allow the child to take the lead as much as possible within the goal of the activity.

Add set phrases to moderate the reactions, e.g., 'never mind', 'it's an accident', 'oh dear', etc.

Discuss real and imagined consequences, e.g., feeling angry when a toy is broken or lost, feeling bullied when her counter is accidentally moved by another player. Moderate 'it's not fair' type responses through discussion and awareness that it's the same for other children some of the time.

Work towards solutions that encourage accepting that nothing can be done, e.g., may involve playing with something else, waiting until later to fix something, etc.

Draw solutions and include 'sometimes accidents happen' as a key phrase.

Discuss at least two more accidents and write down strategies to cope with each situation.

Refer to emotion changes on emotions ladders.

Record a summary or sketch of one of the accidents and the solutions in the child's Book of Feelings under the matching emotion/section of the book.

Role-reversal

Present a scenario and ask the child to suggest an accident and then to suggest a solution.

Meta-challenge

Role-play a scenario where one child over-reacts to the accident, will not listen to the solutions, and cannot be calmed. Discuss the impact on the child and for everyone in the story.

If the child volunteers information relating to their experience of accidents add to the ISCP and use in SUSI 3.3 and explain that you will work on this in a future session.

SCIP Phase 2: SUSI 3

Resource

SUSI 3.2 Understanding unplanned change

Activity 1 Resource: Understanding and coping with accidents

This activity is aimed at helping the child understand vocabulary associated with accidents, making mistakes, and associated feelings.

When presenting the scenario, start by talking about the feelings of the person who caused the accident before talking about the feelings of the person who was hurt or upset by the accident.

Draw these scenarios on a sheet of paper leaving at least half the page blank.

In all pictures, add a moderating adult or child who is observing the scene and can offer solutions. Leave space above this person's head to add thinking bubbles.

Start talking about the first picture and explain that sometimes people make mistakes and have accidents.

❖ breaking something belonging to someone else
❖ spilling a drink on your dinner
❖ breaking a window with a ball
❖ hurting someone when you throw the ball too hard
❖ books falling in a puddle
❖ losing the dice or counters in a game
❖ the dice hits and moves your counter in a board game
❖ spilling something on your clothes
❖ forgetting your friend's birthday
❖ forgetting your lines in the school play

For older children, use idiomatic language to describe accidents and upsets: no need to cry over spilt milk, it's not a big deal, you have to break eggs to make an omelette, etc.

Sample script

"Sometimes things go wrong by accident. Usually, people feel upset when they have an accident. It is just a mistake, and we need to fix it if we can. We can apologise and then get on with something else. It's OK, accidents happen, not to worry".

Adult: "Look what's happened here. Cameron was playing with Ben's car and the wheel has come off. Cameron didn't want to break Ben's car. It was an accident. Cameron is upset because he broke Ben's car. Ben will be upset too. They both like playing with the car".

Draw Ben with an upset face looking at his broken car.

Adult: "Cameron needs to explain and say sorry. Cameron will say, 'It was an accident, I was playing, and the wheel came off. I didn't mean it. I can help you fix it'".

Adult: "Ben will say, 'Never mind, it's OK. I know that it was an accident. It is an old car. The wheel comes off when I play with it too. Dad can fix it'".

Adult: "What will Cameron say?" "That's right, he will say, thank you and sorry".

SCIP Phase 2: SUSI 3

SUSI 3.2 Understanding unplanned change

Activity 2: Understanding and coping with unplanned change

Purpose and target

To help the child understand vocabulary and concepts to describe unplanned change.

Materials

Scenarios and vocabulary from the Activity 2 Resource.
Emotions ladders and child's Book of Feelings from SUSI 2.

Procedure

As in Activity 1, start talking about the first picture and explain that sometimes things happen that were not planned or were not wanted. We have to just say, 'OK, that's the way it is'.

Draw each event on the sheet of paper using speech and thought bubbles and adding feelings and emotion vocabulary the child knows.

Allow the child to take the lead as much as possible within the goal of the activity.

Add set phrases to moderate reactions, e.g., 'never mind', 'there's nothing we can do', 'we have to give up on that for today'. Refer back to the need to be flexible from work in SUSI 3.1.

Discuss 'it's not fair' type responses and develop awareness that it's the same for other children when these things happen.

Work towards solutions that may involve doing something else to distract attention and make the best of a challenging situation.

Draw out the solutions and include "sometimes things just happen" as a title.

Discuss at least two more examples of unplanned change and write down strategies to cope with each situation.

Refer to emotion changes on emotions ladders.

Record a summary or sketch of one of the situations and the solutions in the child's Book of Feelings under the matching emotion/section of the book

Role-reversal

Present a scenario and ask the child to suggest an unplanned change and then to suggest a solution.

Meta-challenge

Role-play a scenario where one child over-reacts to the unplanned change, will not listen to the solutions, and cannot be calmed. Discuss the impact on the child and for everyone in the story.

If the child volunteers information relating to their experience of unplanned change add to the ISCP and use in SUSI 3.3 and explain that you will work on this in a future session.

SCIP Phase 2: SUSI 3
Resource

SUSI 3.2 Understanding unplanned change

Activity 2 Resource: Understanding and coping with unplanned change

This activity is designed to teach vocabulary associated with changes that are outside the adult's control. When presenting the scenario, explain that everyone is surprised/worried/disappointed by the change, including the adults, but there is nothing anyone can do. The only solution is to find an alternative.

Draw these scenarios on a sheet of paper leaving at least half the page blank.

In all pictures, add a moderating adult or child who is observing the scene and can offer solutions. Leave space above this person's head to add thinking bubbles.

Start talking about the first picture and explain that sometimes things happen that can't be easily fixed:

- ❖ the queue for the ride at the funfair is too long
- ❖ the child is too small to go on the ride they like
- ❖ the show at the theatre is sold out
- ❖ there are no strawberries in the shop
- ❖ your friend is ill and can't come to your party
- ❖ your train is delayed, and you have to wait in the station
- ❖ it's too wet to play outside
- ❖ the snow is melting and won't make a good snowman
- ❖ the DVD is scratched and won't play
- ❖ a new toy doesn't work and has to be returned to the shop

SCIP Phase 2: SUSI 3

SUSI 3.2 Understanding unplanned change

Activity 3: Winning and losing a game

Purpose and target

To help the child understand the vocabulary and concepts to describe unplanned change in games and social interactions.

Materials

Emotions ladders and child's Book of Feelings from SUSI 2.

Picture of two or three children playing a board game.

A simple board game, e.g., Snail's Pace Race with no 'jeopardy' squares, e.g., miss a turn.

Cards with 'miss a turn, go back one square and have another turn' written on to add.

Procedure

Introduce the activity by talking about the children playing a board game and discuss how the game is progressing. Explain that the children are taking turns, moving their counters around the board and that the game ends when one person crosses the finish line. Explain that there are special squares to have another turn or go backwards or miss a turn. Explain how these squares impact on the players' feelings. Say, "This boy has just had an extra turn, he feels happy. This girl has to miss a turn, she feels sad, but that's what happens in this game".

Explain how to play the Snail's Pace Race game and that there are no jeopardy or bonus squares so the person who scores highest on the dice will win. It is a game of luck. To make sure he is the winner, you are going to give him two turns every time you have one. Explain that sometimes it's important to let people win so they feel happy.

Play the game allowing the child to cross the line first and discuss how it feels to win and lose.

Play again and explain that this time you will play by the usual rules, i.e., one turn each.

After every turn discuss how everyone is feeling and add set phrases to moderate the reactions, e.g., 'never mind', 'oh dear', 'maybe you'll score higher next time', 'I'm lucky with the scores today', etc.

Teach phrases to accept the dice throws: 'luck of the dice', 'be lucky next time', etc.

Moderate 'it's not fair' type responses through discussion and awareness that it's the same for everyone when they play dice games.

Play through a few times to show the impact of dice on the outcome.

Before starting a new game ask the child if you can include a bonus square, e.g., have another turn. Play and discuss as before.

Repeat with a jeopardy square but agree with the child before the game starts to show that you both agree to take a chance on this making you more or less likely to win.

Refer to emotion changes on emotions ladders for each game.

Record a summary or sketch of winning and losing and the solutions in the child's Book of Feelings under the matching emotion/section of the book.

Meta-challenge

Include a rule change halfway through, e.g., that all red squares mean move ahead one square. Discuss the impact on the child and for everyone in the game when rules are changed in the middle of the game.

SCIP Phase 2: SUSI 3

SUSI 3.3 Making changes in personal routines

Activity 1: Understanding the impact of being flexible

Purpose and target

To help the child understand the impact of being flexible on his own and other people's thoughts and feelings; to help him to be able to reflect on his own flexibility.

Materials

Select a few scenarios from the SUSI 3.1 Resources that are close to the child's own preferred routines and experiences but not exactly the same. You will need to gather information from the child's ISCP or from parent and teacher reports.

Emotions ladders and the child's Book of Feelings from SUSI 2.

Procedure

Say, "Sometimes if people have to change a routine that they like, they will feel upset and sometimes they might feel angry". Point to these feelings on the emotions ladders. Talk about what happens to feelings when a routine is changed, e.g., he feels worried when he doesn't know what will happen.

Start with the first event and draw a conclusion to the event that shows the person becoming upset, angry, shouting, lying on the floor, repeating the same words, or asking the same questions repeatedly. Include the child's typical reaction to a change to his preferred routine in this story.

Discuss thoughts, feelings, and words for all characters starting with the person who is upset by the change. Draw these out on a sheet of paper using speech and thought bubbles and adding emotion vocabulary the child knows.

Explain that this is called being inflexible and say, "This person is upset now and needs to find a way to get back to feeling OK not happy, just OK".

Emphasise that an 'OK ending' is one where you can accept what has happened and can think about it for a little while and feel the upset for a little while, but then you say, "OK, it's not perfect, but it's OK. I can be flexible about this".

Draw this out: The event, the change, the feelings, a pause to feel these feelings (e.g., "have five minutes to feel disappointed") before doing something to feel calmer. Add icons to show things that help the person feel calm (three deep breaths, a stretch, a hug, favourite toys, or being with a pet, etc.). Include ideas from the parent and teacher report on what helps the child to feel calm.

When the impact of the upset has been documented say, "Let's look at how the other people in this story feel" and draw the impact of being flexible on the other people and on the situation. Review the possible solutions to this change to the routine and engage the child as much as possible in the discussion and in providing solutions.

Use the child's own words and write these down in the story for each of the characters. Refer to the emotions ladders and the Book of Feelings to talk about strategies to feel calm.

SCIP Phase 2: SUSI 3

SUSI 3.3 Making changes in personal routines

Activity 2: Understanding the impact of being flexible (personalised)

Purpose and target

To help the child understand the impact of being flexible on his own and other people's thoughts and feelings; to help him to be able to reflect on his own flexibility when unplanned changes happen.

Materials

Blank cards to illustrate child's own experiences as a story sequence.

Pens for child to add his own perspective to the story sequence.

Emotions ladders and child's Book of Feelings from SUSI 2.

Examples of preferred routines and reactions from the child's ISCP.

Procedure

This activity needs to be sensitively managed, preferably when a strong alliance has been established and the child is robust enough to cope with accepting a change. Sufficient time and an appropriate location should be allocated for this work, which will include discussion and practice of calming strategies.

Following from Activity 1 explain that "Today we are going to think about times when your routines are interrupted. Mum told me that you always drive to school, but that sometimes there are red lights on the route, and you feel a bit upset. Let's draw that story".

Illustrate the scenes and add thoughts, feelings, and words for each character. Allow the child to take the lead as much as possible within the goal of the activity. The child should have his own pens and be asked to draw feelings and write in the thinking and speech bubbles. This can provide insights into the child's reasons for adhering to the routine and help identify acceptable solutions.

At each point, discuss a variety of triggers as well as the existing one for the child.

Refer to the emotions ladders throughout.

Discuss each trigger in depth from the child's point of view and work towards a solution and some degree of acceptance.

Explore real and imagined consequences, e.g., coming in a different door when late to school, signing the late register, getting in trouble with the teacher, missed playtime, won't know what to do, etc.

Use set phrases 'never mind', and 'I'm sorry I'm late because …' to moderate the child's emotional response.

Use role-play to teach steps to cope: apologise and explain; ask "what do I need to do now?".

Draw solutions and include 'it's OK to be late sometimes'.

Remind the child that these events are common, and solutions are possible, "everyone is late sometimes", "OK, it's not perfect, but it's OK. I can be flexible".

Record a summary or sketch of a change to routine and the solutions in the child's Book of Feelings under the matching emotion/section of the book.

SCIP Phase 2 | **SUSI 4 Intervention content table**

SUSI 4 Understanding thoughts and intentions of others

SUSI 4 Information

SUSI 4.1 Signalling feelings and intentions (non-verbal)

1 Using eye gaze and body position to signal thoughts and intentions

2 Using non-verbal behaviours to signal boredom and interest

SUSI 4.2 Predicting thoughts and intentions

1 Understanding multiple social context cues plus Resource

2 Understanding multiple social context cues (personalised)

SUSI 4.3 Understanding mismatch of language and thoughts

1 Understanding lies plus Resource

2 Understanding white lies plus Resource

SUSI 4.4 Understanding complex intentions

1 Understanding tricks plus Resource

2 Understanding persuasion plus Resource

SCIP Phase 2: SUSI 4

Information

SUSI 4 Understanding thoughts and intentions of others

The purpose of this Section is to help your child understand social motives and intentions communicated through non-verbal and verbal means. Work in this Section builds on previous strategies to read the social meaning of non-verbal signals to work out the thoughts, feelings, and intentions of others in SUSI 1 and 2. The emphasis is on how multiple cues in social situations can be used to make predictions about upcoming events, thoughts, feelings, and intentions for the characters in the pictures. This is an important skill for social interaction. Understanding multiple social cues in interactions supports the development of shared knowledge between people and is an important skill for the development of reciprocal relationships and friendships.

Work in this Section develops your child's understanding of the mismatch between language and thought. Specifically, concepts are taught to understand and manage hidden intentions, indirect requests, and the subtle use of language for a specific intention. Strategies are taught to recognise and cope with deception, tricks, persuasion, and hints.

Once your child has understood that a mismatch between language and thought exists for specific purposes, recent actual experiences in his/her life will be used to enable your child to understand his/her own social interactions and to being able to resolve upsets and misunderstandings.

How you can help

Teaching in this Section can be tailored to meet your child's needs. Please provide information from your child's recent actual experiences when they found it hard to read social cues in a given situation. The teaching can incorporate working on understanding the social motives that your child needs to understand, e.g., persuasion, tricks. Activities will be developed to use similar social contexts to support your child to generalise this understanding and support strategies to everyday life.

When your child has developed some understanding of these skills you can play simple games that require understanding and sending non-verbal messages. You can set up a range of opportunities for your child to pick up on and use hints. By carefully selecting a suitable treat, you can engage your child in using persuasion to change your mind. You will be advised on key words or phrases that will help your child recognise and respond to the hidden social motive. You will be supported to use role-reversal to model using verbal and non-verbal cues related to hidden intentions and gradually invite your child to use more subtle signals.

SCIP Phase 2: SUSI 4

SUSI 4.1 Signalling feelings and intentions (non-verbal)

Activity 1: Using eye gaze and body position to signal thoughts and intentions

Purpose and target

To enhance the child's awareness of the social meanings carried by non-verbal behaviour such as eye gaze and body position.

Materials

Picture cards to represent conversation topics, e.g., selected from Schubi Combimage cards or similar.

Procedure

Explain the task as follows, "Today we are going to practise talking about different events and topics. I will start and then I will look at one of the other topics. When I look at a new card this means that I want to start a new topic. I won't say, 'I want to talk about the new topic', I will show you that I want to switch topic by looking at the new card. You need to watch me carefully to see how it works".

Lay out four topic cards on the table and start a conversation using one.

Get the conversation going and as the child is talking, turn your gaze to one of the other cards.

Prompt him to notice that you have done this, if necessary, by, e.g., not replying to his contribution, or directly stating, "I want to talk about something else now. Which one am I looking at?"

Repeat with a new set of cards and reduce the verbal prompts by pausing silently and waiting for the child to follow your eye gaze to the new card.

Discuss that he worked out that you wanted to stop talking about X and start talking about Y, because he could see that you were looking away/at something else.

Draw attention to the fact that you didn't say 'I want to talk about Y', but that you were able to signal this intention by just looking.

Make explicit links to thoughts and feelings throughout this activity.

Draw a detailed step-by-step sequence to illustrate what happened; the initial conversation topic, looking and looking away at something else, and the new topic. Illustrate the desire to change the topic in a thought bubble and draw one person looking at the other and observing his/her eye gaze and thinking about the new topic as a result.

SCIP Phase 2: SUSI 4

SUSI 4.1 Signalling feelings and intentions (non-verbal)

Activity 2: Using non-verbal behaviours to signal boredom and interest

Purpose and target

To enhance the child's awareness of the social meanings (boredom and interest) carried by non-verbal behaviour such as eye gaze, facial expression, and body position.

Materials

Picture cards to represent conversation topics, e.g., selected from Schubi Combimage cards.

Pictures of bored and interested faces.

Procedure

Explain that today we are thinking about how we know when someone is interested or bored by what is happening. Model a bored face and show the child the matching picture; repeat with interested expression and picture.

Explain that usually people don't say "I'm bored now", but that we can work out that they feel bored by looking for clues from the person's face, body, and in what is said.

Go on to describe that the clues will be found on the person's face, in her voice, and that she might turn away or give one-word answers. Today we are looking for clues on the person's face.

Start chatting about one of the topics on the cards and ask the child to watch your face and see if you are interested in the topic or bored.

Ask the child to hold up the bored picture when he thinks you are getting bored.

Stop regularly and discuss, e.g., "That's right I was interested, I was looking at you and smiling and saying something".

Or "That's right I was bored. I was looking down/away, and my face was still, and I was looking a bit tired and bored".

Discuss the subtleties of how our faces change when we are bored – flat interaction style, changes in intonation, facial expression, and how much we say.

Repeat with a few more conversations of varying interest to you both.

Role-reversal

Select a topic you know the child is not interested in and begin the conversation.

Ask the child to show interest and then when he has had enough to show a bored face.

Stop to discuss as before and make explicit links to thoughts and intentions throughout this activity.

Discuss solutions when we notice the other person is bored – we should shift to a new topic and talk about something we both like.

Meta-challenge

Repeat with a topic the child is not interested in and begin as before to chat.

When the child shows he has had enough and is showing a bored face, keep talking and ignore the cues. Keep the conversation going through monologue.

Discuss how the child feels when you ignore that he is bored and what he could do in this situation.

SCIP Phase 2: SUSI 4

SUSI 4.2 Predicting thoughts and intentions

Activity 1: Understanding multiple social context cues

Purpose and target

To help the child to identify and describe expected future events, emotions, and thoughts for a variety of characters in complex social situations.

Materials

Pictures of complex social contexts that require understanding of more than one cue (e.g., Winslow Colorcards: Skills for Daily Living: Social Behaviour cards).

Activity 1 Resource.

Plain white cards for drawing predicted events.

Speech bubble and arrow sticky notes to draw attention to cues.

Emotions ladders from SUSI 2 work.

Procedure

Refer to the sample script in the Activity 1 Resource for ideas on what to say for each scene.

Present one picture and describe it, explaining the clues in the picture that indicate what is happening.

Make explicit links to facial expressions and behaviours and refer to the child's emotions ladders as you work and use emotion vocabulary the child knows.

Engage the child in working out the cues as much as possible.

Ask "What might he say?" and record this in a speech bubble.

Ask "What might he think?" and record this in a thought bubble.

Explain how the clues help you to work out what will happen next, what people are thinking, and how the people feel.

Draw the predicted events on the white card and as you add details, repeat how you know this will probably happen.

Repeat with a few scenarios, gradually allowing the child to contribute more as he becomes able to detect the social context cues.

Repeat to reinforce understanding and develop reasoning explicitly.

Emphasise that it is important to consider what all the people in the situation are thinking, feeling, and doing before we can predict.

Meta-challenge

To reinforce the need to consider all positions, make predictions by only looking at part of a scene, cover it up if needed, or make a prediction as soon as you look at the picture and explain this as the cues coming from one person only. Encourage the child to correct you to look at cues from all the people present.

SCIP Phase 2: SUSI 4

Resource

SUSI 4.2 Predicting thoughts and intentions

Activity 1 Resource: Understanding multiple social context cues

This activity is designed to describe how multiple cues in social situations can be combined to make predictions about upcoming events, thoughts, feelings, and intentions for the characters in the pictures.

Select these scenarios from the Winslow Colorcards: Skills for Daily Living: Social Behaviour cards, or use an equivalent scene.

- ❖ dinner guests arrive at a house with a bottle of wine
- ❖ someone using a personal stereo too loudly on a train
- ❖ there is luggage on the seat on a bus
- ❖ one child is inside while the others are playing outside
- ❖ mum is cross about an untidy bathroom
- ❖ a man is opening the door for a woman pushing a pram
- ❖ someone gives the dog a bowl of water on a hot day

Start talking about the picture and explain that you know it is a dinner party because you can see the dining table through the window. It is set for dinner with plates and cutlery and wine glasses and candles. It might be a special occasion. Draw or write dinner party on a sticky arrow and stick it onto the picture.

Sample script

Say, "Now look at these two people. They are standing inside the open door. They have opened the door to let their friends in. These people live here. I know they live here because they have opened the door. They are holding out their arms, they are showing that they are pleased to see their guests. They will give them a hug. They know each other well and they are probably friends".

Say, "Look at these two people, they are walking up the path, they are visiting their friends. They are holding a bottle of wine and waving. They are excited. They have come to celebrate something with their friends. What kind of celebration is it? Are there any clues? Is there a cake on the table? No, then it might not be a birthday. What else might it be?"

SCIP Phase 2: SUSI 4

SUSI 4.2 Predicting thoughts and intentions

Activity 2: Understanding multiple social context cues (personalised)

Purpose and target

To help the child to identify and describe expected future events, emotions, and thoughts for recent personal experiences.

Materials

Ideas for situations the child has experienced but which are not problematic from the ISCP or from recent comments from parents or teachers.

Speech bubble and arrow sticky notes.

Emotions ladders from SUSI 2 work.

Procedure

Following from Activity 1 explain, "Last time we were working out what people might be thinking and saying. We were looking for clues to work out what might happen next. Let's see if you can work out what is going to happen in these stories about your class/family".

Draw simple pictures to represent the child's recent social experiences in school and at home. **These should not be challenging situations.** For example, draw a group of children holding different toys as indicators of their preferred activity for playtime.

Refer to the first scene, "Here are your friends, Kimran, Lily, and Morgan. They are holding their favourite toys. Kimran wants to play with her dolls. Tell me what Lily wants to do and what Morgan wants to play".

Discuss and role-play what each child might think or say.

Say, "These children want to play different things".

Explain how the clues help you to work out what will happen next, what people are thinking, and how the people feel.

Draw the predicted events on the white card and as you add details, repeat how you know this will probably happen.

Repeat with a few scenarios, gradually allowing the child to contribute more as he becomes able to detect the social context cues.

Repeat to reinforce understanding and develop reasoning explicitly.

Emphasise that it is important to consider what all the people in the situation are thinking, feeling, and doing before we can predict.

Role-reversal

Draw only the people in a recent experience and ask the child to add to the drawing with thought and speech bubbles and to explain the situation. Support with details from the ISCP as needed.

SCIP Phase 2: SUSI 4

SUSI 4.3 Understanding mismatch of language and thoughts

Activity 1: Understanding lies

Purpose and target

To help the child understand the concept of lies and the purpose they serve; to develop the child's understanding of and ability to manage complex personal situations.

Materials

Examples of situations and lies from the Activity 1 Resource.

Speech bubble sticky notes.

Emotions ladders from SUSI 2 work.

Procedure

Teach the meaning of true and false by sorting very obvious statements related to things the child will be sure about, e.g., your name is Mary.

Select an example from Activity 1 Resource, e.g., a boy dropping a cup and it breaks.

Draw thought bubbles and write "Oh no, Mum will be cross" and "I don't want to get into trouble".

Draw a speech bubble and write "I didn't drop the cup".

Tell the child this is not true; it is a lie.

Discuss why the boy said this and explain that we tell lies for all kinds of reasons – to play tricks, tell jokes, get out of trouble, and make ourselves appear brave or clever.

Explain that this boy knows Mum will be cross, so he wants to get out of trouble.

Provide other words for lies as needed.

Repeat with other lies from the Activity 1 Resource and discuss different reasons why someone might tell a lie, e.g., to cheat or show off.

Repeat with a few scenarios, gradually allowing the child to contribute more as he becomes able to detect the lies and understand the reasons.

Refer to the emotions ladders throughout.

Role-reversal

Present a scenario to the child and explain that this child wants to show off to a friend, and ask the child to suggest a lie he could tell.

Explain that lies are not the best way to interact with our friends and discuss the consequences of lying and what people will think of someone who tells lies.

SCIP Phase 2: SUSI 4

Resource

SUSI 4.3 Understanding mismatch of language and thoughts

Activity 1 Resource: Understanding lies

This activity is designed to enable the child to understand and describe a complex scenario involving lies and to understand the consequences of lying.

Draw these scenarios on a sheet of paper leaving at least half the page blank and use the following lies as examples.

A child in class who didn't do her homework

- ❖ "I left my homework at home"
- ❖ "Mum took my homework to work with her by mistake"
- ❖ "the dog ate my homework"
- ❖ "I've got my brother's school bag and he has mine"

Someone breaking something

- ❖ "the dog tripped me and broke the cups"
- ❖ "I didn't play with the train today"

Cheating at a game

- ❖ moving more places on the board than the dice showed
- ❖ lying about the dice score
- ❖ saying the ball was in/out in football
- ❖ saying you made it home in Rounders

Drawing and writing your name on the walls with a pen

- ❖ "my pen slipped and went all over the wall"
- ❖ "it wasn't me"

Don't want to share a toy

- ❖ "you can play with it later"
- ❖ "I have to go home now for my lunch"
- ❖ "my Mum says you can't have a go"
- ❖ "you wouldn't like it"
- ❖ "it's not for little boys"

Showing off for our friends

- ❖ "I'm allowed to stay up until 10.00 p.m."
- ❖ exaggerate the amount of pocket money received
- ❖ "I'm allowed to watch the Harry Potter films by myself"

SCIP Phase 2: SUSI 4

Activity 2: Understanding white lies

Purpose and target

To help the child understand the concept of white lies and the purpose they serve in complex personal situations.

Materials

Examples of situations and white lies from the Activity 2 Resource.

Speech bubble and thought bubble sticky notes.

Emotions ladders and child's Book of Feelings from SUSI 2 work.

Procedure

Explain that sometimes people don't say exactly what they are thinking. They might tell a lie, but they tell the lie for a good reason. The reason is so as not to hurt someone's feelings.

Present a scenario from the Activity Resource and explain that we can work out what the people can say so as not to upset the other people in the stories.

Present a picture of a boy opening a present. Explain that it is his birthday and he wants a remote-control car, but his Granny has given him Dr Who pyjamas.

Work through the sample script as described in the Activity 2 Resource to show the impact of telling the truth and the impact of the white lie on Granny's feelings.

Explore solutions to get what he wants, e.g., he might be able to ask his Mum for what he really wants, he can save up, he can ask for this gift for Christmas, etc.

Add the positives of the gift for the boy, e.g., they are his favourite TV character.

Add a sketch of this to the child's Book of Feelings under disappointment.

Repeat with different scenarios and support the child to make contributions to the drawings and the white lies.

Discuss explicitly that the words and thoughts don't match and that this is important so as not to hurt the other person.

Role-reversal

Present a scenario and ask the child to suggest a white lie he could tell to avoid hurting someone's feelings. Support as needed.

Meta-challenge

Present a scenario and tell the truth which will hurt someone's feelings, e.g., I don't want Dr Who pyjamas.

Discuss what will happen and ask the child to suggest a white lie he could tell to avoid hurting someone's feelings. Support as needed.

Record a summary or sketch of a white lie in the child's Book of Feelings under the matching emotion/section of the book.

SCIP Phase 2: SUSI 4

Resource

SUSI 4.3 Understanding mismatch of language and thoughts

Activity 2 Resource: Understanding white lies

Draw these scenarios on a sheet of paper leaving at least half the page blank.

A boy opens a present from his grandmother, but he doesn't like it

- ❖ "thank you very much"
- ❖ "I really like Dr Who, thank you"
- ❖ "I need some new pyjamas; my old ones are too short"

A friend wants you to play a game, but you really don't like it

- ❖ "I don't know how to play that game. Can we play something else?"

Auntie suggests a trip to the Zoo. You don't want to go

- ❖ "thanks Auntie, the Zoo is great, but I went last week with a friend"

Mum buys a new dress; you think the colours are ugly

- ❖ "you will look pretty at the party, Mum"

Someone invites you to a party, but you don't want to go

- ❖ "I think we are going to my Granny's that day"
- ❖ "I will need to check with Mum"

Someone reads you a story they have written. You don't like it

- ❖ "that is a really interesting and complicated story"
- ❖ "I liked the character who lived in the barn"

Sample script

Start talking about the boy's birthday. His preferred present is a remote-control car. Add a thought bubble above his head and write, 'I want a remote-control car'. Add Granny's thoughts: 'Dylan loves Dr Who' and 'He needs some new pyjamas'.

Say, "Here is Granny and here is Dylan. It is Dylan's birthday. Granny has a present for him. Dylan hopes it is a remote-control car".

Ask the child to look at Granny's thoughts and ask the child to work out what the present is, i.e., Dr Who pyjamas. Say, "What will Dylan think when he opens the present?" "That's right he will think, 'It's not a remote-control car'".

Draw the boy looking at the present but leave the facial expression blank. Write "it's not a remote-control car" in a thinking bubble and ask the child to draw the facial expression.

Name this feeling as disappointed and refer to the emotions ladders and Book of Feelings.

Draw the boy holding the pyjamas and add the thought 'I didn't want pyjamas'.

Stop here and discuss with child what he should say now.

Draw the boy saying, "I didn't want pyjamas". Draw Grandma and explore her thoughts and feelings on hearing this.

Explain to the child that this is a time when people sometimes tell a "white lie".

Explain that this is something we say so that we don't hurt someone's feelings.

Add the white lie as "Thank you Grandma – I like the pyjamas". Use a different colour speech bubble sticky note if necessary to indicate the white lie.

Draw Grandma as feeling happy and contrast with her feeling upset when the boy said, "I didn't want pyjamas".

SCIP Phase 2: SUSI 4

SUSI 4.4 Understanding complex intentions

Activity 1: Understanding tricks

Purpose and target

To help the child understand the concept of tricks and the mismatch between language and thought so that he develops strategies to cope with complex personal situations.

Materials

Examples of tricks from the Activity 1 Resource.

Speech bubble sticky notes.

Emotions ladder and Book of Feelings from SUSI 2 work.

Procedure

Explain that sometimes people don't say exactly what they are thinking. They might tell a lie, but they tell the lie for fun. The reason is to make someone laugh. This is called a trick. A trick is when you get someone to believe something that isn't true. It can be funny when you trick someone.

Work through the examples in the Activity Resource.

Draw simple pictures to represent a simple trick between two children, e.g., A boy points to the girl's foot and says, "Careful, your shoelace is undone!".

Look at these pictures and discuss what the trick is, i.e., her shoelace is not undone. Discuss why the boy would say this, and if it is a funny trick or a nasty trick.

Discuss the boy and say he wants to play a trick on the girl. He wants the girl to believe that what he says is true. He wants her to 'fall for' his trick.

Describe what will happen when the girl looks at her shoes; the boy will say, "I tricked you".

Make explicit reference to the vocabulary, i.e., "that's a trick", "she fell for it", etc.

Repeat the same trick but this time, don't fall for it, and say, "You're only saying that because you want me to think my shoe is open. It's only a trick. I'm not going to fall for it again". Say, "Thanks for telling me", but don't look or fix it. Move away.

Explain that if your shoe is open, you should tie it up so as not to fall, so it is important to know.

Repeat with different scenarios and support the child to make contributions to the drawings.

Emphasise key vocabulary from the Activity 1 Resource.

Say, "Sometimes tricks can be funny. When we fall for a trick, we feel embarrassed and silly, and the other person will laugh".

Explain how to check with someone you trust if you are suspicious of a trick being played.

Play a simple trick on the child from those listed in the Activity Resource and discuss how it feels.

Repeat, this time showing a clear facial expression that it is a trick and discuss.

Record a summary or sketch of a trick in the child's Book of Feelings under the matching emotion/section of the book.

Role-reversal

Ask the child to act out tricking you with the same or new ideas.

SCIP Phase 2: SUSI 4
Resource

SUSI 4.4 Understanding complex intentions

Activity 1 Resource: Understanding tricks

This activity is designed to enable the child to describe a complex scenario involving tricks and to develop strategies to cope.

Draw these scenarios on a sheet of paper leaving at least half the page blank:

Simple tricks

a boy points to the girl's foot and says, "Careful, your shoelace is undone!"

a boy looks/points behind the girl and says, "Here comes your Mum"

Tricks that cause disappointment/fear

"there's pizza for lunch today. We get to add our own toppings"

a boy points to the girl's hair and makes a scared face, and says, "Watch out there's a spider in your hair!"

Tricks that might get you into trouble in school

❖ one boy says to another, "There's no football after school today. You can go home with your brother"

❖ "Teacher said we don't have to do any homework tonight"

❖ at playtime, someone tells you to go inside as the teacher wants to give you a certificate

❖ "Mr Smith, the Headteacher, wants to see you in his office"

Examples of associated vocabulary and phrases

Believe.

Trust.

Suspicious.

Doubtful.

Made you look, made you stare.

Fooled you.

You fell for it.

Made you scream, made you shout, made you look all about.

You're so silly. We're not allowed in the school kitchen/science lab.

I got you into trouble.

SCIP Phase 2: SUSI 4

SUSI 4.4 Understanding complex intentions

Activity 2: Understanding persuasion

Purpose and target

To help the child understand the concept of persuasion and understand how to give good reasons for things he wants to happen.

Materials

Examples of situations from the Activity 2 Resource.

Plain paper and speech bubble and thought bubble sticky notes.

Two or three play people or laminated figures of adults, boys, and girls.

Emotions ladder and Book of Feelings from SUSI 2 work.

Procedure

Explain that sometimes people want us to do something and when we don't want to do it, they will keep asking and will give some good reasons why we should do it. This is called persuading you to do something.

Work through the examples in the Activity Resource.

Draw simple pictures to represent a situation between a Mum and a child, e.g., A mum wants the boy to put his coat on to go outside.

Let's look at these pictures and work out what both people are thinking and what one person wants the other person to do. They will have good reasons and will try to make the other person change their mind.

Take the first scenario and explain both people's thoughts, e.g., for the boy, "I want to play outside, I don't want to wear my coat". Explain Mum's thoughts as "it's too cold to play outside without a coat".

Draw the boy and the Mum at the top of two columns on a sheet of paper.

Draw the Mum's words as she gives good reasons. Put numbers beside the reasons.

Draw the boy's thought bubble showing a change in thinking to "OK, I will wear my coat. It is cold and if I wear my coat I can stay outside for longer".

Add a speech bubble, "OK Mum, you persuaded me to put my coat on".

Repeat with other scenarios and engage the child in suggesting good reasons and what the other person will think when he is persuaded to change his mind.

Emphasise key vocabulary, e.g., persuade, change your mind, listen to the good reasons, agree to think it over, etc.

Role-reversal

Present a scenario for the child to provide good reasons to make one person change their mind. Record a list of good reasons and support as needed to persuade.

Meta-challenge

Show that persuasion doesn't always work by refusing, e.g., to agree to put a coat on, and that the boy then has less time to play outside. Discuss consequences of not listening to the good reasons and how he has to come in earlier because he is cold, but if he had listened to Mum, he would be able to stay out longer.

SCIP Phase 2: SUSI 4

Resource

SUSI 4.4 Understanding complex intentions

Activity 2 Resource: Understanding persuasion

This activity is designed to enable the child to describe a complex scenario involving persuasion and to develop strategies to give, and listen to, good reasons.

Draw these scenarios on a sheet of paper leaving at least half the page blank. Add the good reasons to the discussion sheet as you work.

A mum wants the boy to put his coat on to go outside

❖ you'll catch cold
❖ all the other children have a coat on
❖ you can stay out longer if you wear your coat
❖ it's too cold to play outside without it

A mum wants the boy to eat his vegetables at dinner

❖ carrots are healthy
❖ they are Daddy's favourite
❖ vegetables help you to grow up strong
❖ ten more peas, let's count them

Dad wants you to get ready for bed

❖ it's really late, you've already stayed up for an hour
❖ you need to get up early tomorrow
❖ you can stay up later on Saturday night
❖ you can have two stories tonight

The children want the teacher to cancel homework for tonight

❖ we worked hard today, Miss
❖ we can have homework tomorrow
❖ we had homework yesterday

The teacher wants the group to work harder

- ❖ no playtime unless all work is done
- ❖ we can't go to PE until the room is tidy
- ❖ there will be extra house points for the group who works best

You want ice cream for dessert

- ❖ I will eat all my dinner
- ❖ I will help clear the table
- ❖ I will go to bed on time tonight

More complex situations:

- ❖ a child aged 12 wants to see a 15-certificate film
- ❖ a child wants to buy trainers not suitable for sports
- ❖ a child wants to have their ears pierced
- ❖ a child wants a pet

SCIP Phase 2	SUSI 5 Intervention content table

SUSI 5 Understanding friendship

SUSI 5 Information

SUSI 5.1 Understanding interests in friendship

1 Understanding personal interests

2 Planning a playtime

3 Trying new interests

4 Planning a playtime (personalised)

SUSI 5.2 Understanding the impact of preferred interests

1 Identifying a preferred interest

2 The impact of preferred interests on friendship

3 The impact of preferred interests on friendship (personalised)

4 Understanding fantasy and reality plus Resource

5 The impact of fantasy worlds

SUSI 5.3 Understanding friendship skills

1 Friendship role-play

2 Identifying and solving problems in friendship

3 Identifying and solving problems in friendship (personalised)

4 Understanding friendship (personalised)

SCIP Phase 2: SUSI 5

Information

SUSI 5 Understanding friendship

The purpose of this Section is to help your child understand the role of interests in building and maintaining friendships and how preferred interests can impact on a friendship. Your child will reflect on what he likes to do and consider whether others' interests are the same as theirs or not. The importance of shared interests in making new friends is included. Work in this Section uses role-play to enhance your child's ability to ask questions to find a shared interest. Your child will be taught how to plan a play date based on shared interests so that both people will enjoy the playtime. Your child will be able to talk about interests and favourite activities for themselves and his/her friends. The benefits of joining in with new games is covered.

Vocabulary is introduced to understand a preferred interest and the impact it can have on friendship. There will be times when your child cannot follow his own preference, so problem-solving and calming strategies are revised. This Section will refer back to work completed in SUSI 2 on emotions to understand friendships. The link between feeling left out and not wanting to try new things is explained.

Vocabulary and concepts linked to fantasy and reality are taught to understand the impact of fantasy worlds on learning and friendship.

In general, the emphasis is on learning how to understand and resolve issues that arise commonly in friendship such as sharing, feeling bored, or being left out. Training in how to join in with activities not of his/her choosing and to practise different friendship skills is aimed at learning how to resolve common issues that occur in friendships.

How you can help

Teaching in this Section can be tailored to meet your child's needs. Please provide information from your child's recent actual experiences about peer play and interactions. The teaching can incorporate working on understanding the signs of interest and boredom, turn-taking or sharing that will facilitate improved peer interactions. Activities will be developed to use familiar social contexts to support him to generalise the skills to everyday life. Strategies to resolve friendship issues will be shared with home and school and can be used to prepare your child for an upcoming play event or reflect on a recent playtime. Reflecting on successes is as important as reflecting on upsets for managing friendship skills and peer relations.

When your child has developed some understanding of friendship skills, you can plan play dates by listing everyone's interests and agreeing shared and new interests to try. Role-play and drawings are helpful in preparing for play dates and resolving upsets.

SCIP Phase 2: SUSI 5

SUSI 5.1 Understanding interests in friendship

Activity 1: Shared interests

Purpose and target

To help the child understand the importance of shared interests and asking about people's interests in building friendships.

Materials

Notebook to create a Friendship book.

Pictures of the same few children doing a range of different activities together in different pairings, e.g., from Schubi Combimage, Sentimage, or Tell Me About It sequence sets.

List of interests from the ISCP.

Procedure

Explain that when children are friends they often like doing some of the same things and this is called 'shared interests' and 'having things in common'.

Start by talking about the children in one of the pictures and say, "Here is a picture of Dylan and Jenna at the zoo. They both like animals. Liking animals is a shared interest. It is something they have in common".

Enter a heading, 'Shared Interests', on one page in the Friendship book and draw a table with enough rows and columns to record the children and their interests. In this example, enter Jenna and Dylan and next to both names write 'animals', and explain that this shows that they both like animals.

Now look at another picture with the same two children doing something different and add this interest to the list, e.g., painting.

Emphasise the words 'shared interests' and 'in common'.

Take a new picture with two new children and repeat the discussion of what they like doing together and write their names and their shared interests on the table.

Now suggest other activities that these children might like and repeat the discussion on shared interests, e.g., Jenna likes animals so maybe she will like walking the dog. If you have pictures representing the same children use these as prompts.

Repeat until you have four children with a mixture of shared and not shared interests for this group and discuss what each of the friends could do together and how they might play together and have fun together because they will enjoy the activities.

Include the idea that someone might not want to join in because they don't like the activity and talk about what it would feel like to be left out, i.e., the only one who doesn't want to play or the only one who likes a particular game.

Refer to the emotions ladders if needed and add a short story about shared and not shared interests to the Friendship book.

Personalisation

To help the child understand his interests and favourite activities and how they overlap with others, include some interests for the child you are working with on the table and add his name. Go through each interest identified from the pictures and ask the child to tell you whether he is interested in that activity or not. Add the activities the child is interested in to his column and discuss who from the list he has shared interests with and who he does not.

SCIP Phase 2: SUSI 5

SUSI 5.1 Understanding interests in friendship

Activity 2: Asking about interests

Purpose and target

To help the child understand the importance of shared interests and finding out about people's interests in building friendships.

Materials

List of interests created in Activity 1 in the child's Friendship book.

Child's Friendship book from Activity 1: This activity forms one part of making a Friendship book for use throughout Phase 2.

Emotions ladders of emotion vocabulary created in SUSI 2.

Procedure

Using the list of interests created in Activity 1, add a new child to the table. Explain that this boy is new at school, and we need to ask what he likes so that he can join in and make friends. Explain that we don't know what this child likes to do, but we can find out by asking questions.

Start a role-play and say, "I'll be Dylan and I will ask the new boy what he likes to do". Act both roles.

Ask a question, e.g., "What's your name?", "Do you like animals/football/computer games?", "What do you like to do at the weekend?", etc.

Role-play each question and answer and write all the questions down in the Friendship book on a page headed, 'Asking about other people's interests'.

Encourage the child to join in with thinking of questions and answering for the new boy.

Use the questions to fill in the interests columns on the table, answering with a few new interests.

Role-reversal

Ask the child to find out who likes the same things as the new boy by coming up with questions to ask the existing list of children, e.g., "do you like making up dance routines?".

Role-play the conversation with each child, varying the answers to accept and refuse the offer of joining in with the boy's interests.

As in Activity 1, discuss what each of the friends could do together and how they might play together and who would be left out.

Repeat with another new child and other new interests and support the child to ask questions to determine levels of interest in the group, role-playing as before.

Refer to the emotions ladders if needed and add a short story about shared and not shared interests to the Friendship book.

Personalisation

Find ways to begin to talk to the child about his interests and whether other children like the same thing. Encourage reflecting on his own interests and who has the same interests as him. If the child volunteers that they do not like to try new things explain that this can be discussed in a future session and make a note in Activity 5.

SCIP Phase 2: SUSI 5

SUSI 5.1 Understanding interests in friendship

Activity 3: Understanding personal interests

Purpose and target

To help the child understand his own interests as part of understanding the nature of shared interests in friendship.

Materials

Child's Friendship book from Activity 1: This activity forms one part of making a Friendship book for use throughout Phase 2.

Information on the child's interests from the ISCP.

Procedure

Introduce the task as making a list of what the child likes and what their interests are so that he can plan a play date with a friend and do things they both like.

On a new page in the child's Friendship book add a heading, 'All about me and my interests'.

Explain that it is important to know what we like and what we don't like when we are making friends, e.g., so that we can play games with someone who likes the same games as us, go for pizza together, watch a football match together, etc.

Add a range of questions and answers to the Friendship book e.g.,

How old am I? I am _____ years old

When is my birthday? My birthday is on ___ of _____

My favourite food is: _____, but I don't like:_____

My favourite book is: _____, but I don't like:_____

My favourite game is: _____, but I don't like:_____

My favourite film is: _____, but I don't like:_____

My favourite lesson is: _____, but I don't like:_____

After school I like to: _____, but I don't like:_____

On Saturdays I like to: _____, but I don't like:_____

If necessary, ask the child to complete some sections at home or at playtime with support from parent or school staff as required.

Discuss potential play dates in preparation for Activity 4, e.g., "you like superhero films, so if there was a new film at the cinema, you could ask someone who also likes superheroes to come with you".

Explain that if he asked someone who didn't like superheroes, they probably wouldn't like the film and would feel bored and not have a good time.

SCIP Phase 2: SUSI 5

SUSI 5.1 Understanding interests in friendship

Activity 4: Planning a playtime

Purpose and target

To help the child understand how his interests overlap with others or not and how to discuss interests to plan an enjoyable playtime.

Materials

Child's Friendship book from Activity 1: This activity forms one part of making a Friendship book for use throughout Phase 2.

Pictures of children with/without something to indicate an interest.

Lists of common interests for this child's age range and locality, including any current playground crazes arranged as a set of likes and dislikes for each potential friend.

Procedure

In the child's Friendship book start a new page headed, 'Planning a playtime'.

Start by showing a picture of a child and use a list of interests shared with the child and say, "Let's pretend that this girl is coming to play with you after school. Here is a list of the things she likes: Ten pin bowling, snakes and ladders, art and crafts, bike rides, dogs, swimming. Here are the things that she doesn't like: Reading, science, playing with dolls".

Stick these lists into the child's Friendship book and ask the child to add a tick to the things he likes and a cross for those he doesn't like. If he is unsure, add a question mark.

Explain that the playtime will be fun for both by including things that both children like.

Start to plan the visit by writing a list of all the shared interests. Ask the child to decide which activity would be good to start with and put this first on the list. Keep adding to the list until there are a few shared interests. Add snack and TV time to the list and explain that usually children like to have a snack and that TV might be good for when you feel tired.

Repeat using at least three different children with a range of shared and not shared interests or until the child can confidently detect the shared interests and create the 'plan for playtime'.

Include at least one friend who dislikes at least some of the child's interests and ask, "Is there anything a bit tricky about this visit? What can you do about it?".

Discuss the consequences of suggesting something the new friend doesn't like and how this will impact on the friendship.

Discuss the benefits of trying something new and taking turns to choose what to do.

Provide ideas for general enjoyment and fun as a solution and add a few examples to the child's Friendship book and update the child's list of interests created in Activity 3.

Meta-challenge

Add items to the plan for playtime that the children do not share and discuss what might happen. Engage the child in noticing that this would be difficult for either himself or the new friend and in providing a solution. Present and discuss a child who has only one interest and many dislikes, some of which overlap with the child's interests. Discuss what happens when one person is not interested in many things and what the playtime will be like for both people. Discuss how to join in for a while to try new things and make note of the child's reactions to this for work in Activity 5.

SCIP Phase 2: SUSI 5

SUSI 5.1 Understanding interests in friendship

Activity 5: Trying new interests

Purpose and target

To help the child understand the importance of joining in with activities not of his choosing and develop strategies to show an interest in others.

Materials

Child's Friendship book from Activity 1: This activity forms one part of making a Friendship book for use throughout Phase 2.

Pictures or drawings to support the story, added as you narrate.

Procedure

Following from Activity 4, remind the child that sometimes we 'go along with' what our friends like so that we can join in and have fun and not be left out.

Explain good reasons for joining in and having a go at new things, e.g., you don't know if you will like it, to be friendly and supportive.

On a new page in the child's Friendship book add a heading, 'Trying new things' and draw the following events as you tell a story about one friend who doesn't like football but that his friend is in the final of a competition and wants all his friends to come along to support him on the day.

Explain how important it is to have friends cheering when you are trying very hard to do something. Say, "Even though we don't like football and you've never watched a match before, we can be kind to our friend and give it a try because it is important to him. Let's see what might happen".

In turn, draw and discuss the following scenarios: going to the game and his friend wins, they can celebrate together; going to the game and his friend loses, he can offer support and be kind; staying at home and his friend wins, he is left out of the party to celebrate; staying at home and his friend loses, his friend is upset and crying, and he cannot say kind words and remind him that he did his best.

Include examples of what he could say in these different situations, e.g., "you were brilliant", "you played your best", and the effect of these on his friend's feelings in both the win and lose scenarios.

Repeat with a different example of e.g., playing a new game together that one child has never played before and discuss that he can try, his friend will explain what to do, and that he will need a few turns before he understands what to do and whether he likes it or not.

Discuss the options and implications: say "no" and end up playing alone or be persuaded to have a go and try something new. Explain that trying a new thing might reveal that you do like it, and it becomes a new interest, or not liking it. If you don't like it you can say, "Thank you for asking, I tried it, but I didn't really like it".

Role-play asking for help to understand the rules, having a practice-turn with help, and practising at home to get better at the game for next time.

Refer to the emotions ladders as needed and use emotion vocabulary that the child understands.

Add a short sketch/story about trying new things to the child's Friendship book.

SCIP Phase 2: SUSI 5

SUSI 5.1 Understanding interests in friendship

Activity 6: Planning a playtime (personalised)

Purpose and target

To help the child understand the importance of shared interests and finding out about people's interests in building friendships; the child will be able to ask questions to find a shared interest and use this to play with others.

Materials

Child's Friendship book from Activity 1: This activity forms one part of making a Friendship book for use throughout Phase 2.

List of interests and questions about interests created in Activities 2 and 3.

List of names of children from class and home and some of their interests.

Procedure

Refer back to the list of interests created in Activity 3 and the questions from Activity 2.

Refer the child to Activity 4, planning a playtime, and explain that this time he needs to plan a playtime for him and a new friend from his class.

On a new page in the child's Friendship book add a heading, 'Planning a playtime for me'.

Draw a table with enough rows and columns to record the children and their interests and add the child's name to the first column along with their interests. Add one child's name from the child's friendship circle or class group.

Point out that we don't know what this child likes to do but we can find out what he likes by asking. Show the child the questions created in Activity 2 and start a role-play.

Say, "I'll be the boy in your class, and you can ask me questions to find out what I like. We will write this down under his name". Use the information provided to answer as fully as possible.

Role-play each question and answer and write all the answers down.

Support the child to ask questions that help fill in the columns on the list of interests.

Discuss whether they have anything in common and whether they could play together.

Support the child in role-play to ask a child to play together on a shared interest. As the role-play develops write down or draw what happened in the Friendship book, e.g., "We both like football, I asked him to play, he said yes, we played together, and it was fun".

Throughout this activity discuss with the child the nature of interests, limited interests, and being open to trying new things and why this is helpful in making new friends.

Explain that the child can add to the table in his Friendship book to ask questions of his peers about their interests and use this to plan who to play with and what to do in a playtime.

Throughout this activity refer to each person's emotions using vocabulary the child knows and if needed refer to the emotions ladders created in SUSI 2 work.

Add a few examples of potential playmates to the child's Friendship book and arrange to review after he has had a chance to ask some children about their interests and to play.

SCIP Phase 2: SUSI 5

SUSI 5.2 Understanding the impact of preferred interests

Activity 1: Identifying a preferred interest

Purpose and target

To help the child to understand what his own preferred interests are and the feelings and words associated with them.

Materials

Child's Friendship book from Activity 1: This activity forms one part of making a Friendship book for use throughout Phase 2.

Pictures of e.g., a computer game, a chess board, football players, trains, history books, comic characters, animals, dinosaurs, etc.

Laminated figures of four or five different children, one for each interest.

Procedure

On a new page in the child's Friendship book add a heading, 'My interests'.

Create a list of people and their interests as in Activity 1 by adding a name for each of the new characters at the top of each column and a row for each interest.

Say, "Now, we're going to find out what these children like and whether they can play together, just like we did before".

Start with the first child. Say, "Here is Michael, and he likes trains". Write "trains" next to his name. Support the child to use the questions from Activity 2 to ask questions to the character, to find out what else he likes.

Present the other pictures of interests one at a time. The child will ask, e.g., "do you like history?" The character will reply "no" to all questions.

Add each interest to the subsequent rows as the child asks and mark an X against each interest.

After one or two questions, the character will say, "No, I only like trains, I don't play with anything else".

Continue with one or two more characters and allow the child to join in and begin to complete the list of interests by marking an 'X' when the character replies "no".

When the table is complete, begin to discuss the impact: The children will not be able to play with each other, they might have to play alone.

Discuss the importance of having more than one interest.

Refer to the child's Book of Feelings from SUSI 2 work as needed.

Begin to talk about whether the children could try new things, take turns, and have fun with a friend, e.g., football first, then trains. Refer back to SUSI 5.1 Activity 5 as needed.

Personalisation

Now add another name and add one of the child's preferred interests to the list under the new name. Repeat the questioning role-play and ask the child to answer for the new character. Observe what level of insight the child has regarding his own interests, its impact on friendship, and whether he would try a new thing on the list so as to join in.

SCIP Phase 2: SUSI 5

SUSI 5.2 Understanding the impact of preferred interests

Activity 2: The impact of preferred interests on friendship

Purpose and target

To help the child to understand the impact of his own preferred interests on friendship and loneliness and provide support to try new interests.

Materials

Picture of a child playing on a computer game.
Pictures of a child playing football, a winning team photo, lifting a trophy, a crowd cheering.

Procedure

Refer back to the story in SUSI 5.1 Activity 5 about trying new things and elaborate on the story of the school football team in the final of a football competition, and the teacher has asked all the children in the class to come along to cheer for the team on the day.

Explain that on Saturday, some children are excited to go along to cheer for their team, some will go even though they don't like football very much, and that one child is refusing to go. This child wants to stay at home so he can play his favourite computer game. He has refused to go to the football match. He said he is only interested in one thing. He is not interested in football.

Explain that he stayed at home playing his computer game. He missed the match. He doesn't know the score and doesn't know if his school won or lost the trophy.

At school on Monday there is a special announcement: The football team won the match on Saturday. A journalist is coming to school to take photographs and will write a story for the newspaper. Everyone is really excited.

The football team and the children gather for the photo. This boy doesn't join in for the photo. He stands to watch the celebration and feels left out and lonely.

Discuss that the reason he didn't go was because he wanted to stay at home and play on the computer and that this means he was left out of the fun and the celebrations.

Talk about liking the computer game too much and that this means he was left out.

Refer back to the list of single interests from Activity 1 and explain that this can happen when we have interests that we 'like too much' and when we are not willing to 'try new things'.

Draw pictures to illustrate the boy on his own and looking sad.

Suggest a solution for how to join in at school and say well done to the boys and be in the photo cheering and clapping for the team.

Suggest a solution for next time; draw another story with a different celebration event and the same child being asked to come along and choosing to join in even if only for a while.

Stop and ask the child what the boy should do: should he stay at home because that is what he is interested in, or should he find a way to join in?

Engage the child in role-play as the child who wants to stay home and give good reasons to join in.

Support the child to contribute as much as possible at this point and observe his reactions to the boy not being able to indulge his favourite pastime in preparation for Activity 3.

Add a sketch/story to the child's Friendship book.

SCIP Phase 2: SUSI 5

SUSI 5.2 Understanding the impact of preferred interests

Activity 3: The impact of preferred interests on friendship (personalised)

Purpose and target

To help the child to understand the impact of his preferred interests on joining in with friendship or family activities; to provide support by emphasising the language of joining in and compromise.

Materials

Information from the child's ISCP on preferred interests and the impact of preferred interests on his play and peer interaction.

This activity needs to be sensitively managed, preferably when a strong alliance has been established and the child is robust enough to cope with direct feedback.

Procedure

Following from Activity 2, explain that sometimes the child might not want to join in with events because he would like to stay at home to do his favourite thing. Explain, "I know that you like building with bricks. I know that sometimes you don't want to visit Grandma because you have to stop playing with your bricks. I know that you love to see Grandma and that you like it when she comes to your house, and you can show her what you have made".

Let's draw that in your Friendship book.

Describe each step as you draw and explain the impact on him and the others in the scene, as in Activity 2.

Draw out two different endings: He stays at home and Grandma misses him and is sad; he goes and sees Grandma and can tell her what he has made, and she is pleased to see him.

Suggest that he can ask Mum to take photos of his building to show Grandma, or take some bricks to Grandma's house as a compromise.

The aim of this is to raise self-awareness. Do not press for change in this activity, but do present options for changes that would make it 'OK for everyone'.

SCIP Phase 2: SUSI 5

SUSI 5.2 Understanding the impact of preferred interests

Activity 4: Understanding fantasy and reality

Purpose and target

To enhance the child's understanding of vocabulary and concepts linked to fantasy and reality and become aware of fantasy elements in his own conversation.

Materials

Child's Friendship book from Activity 1: This activity forms one part of making a Friendship book for use throughout Phase 2.

Sorting labels written on cards e.g., Real, Fact, Fiction, Imaginary, and Not real.

Vocabulary for real and imaginary as listed in the Activity 4 Resource, written on single cards.

Pictures of real people and objects and fictional/fantasy characters and objects.

Short scripts based in reality and fantasy scripts from the Activity 4 Resource.

Procedure

Present the labels to represent fantasy and reality and explain that the child must sort the cards and decide whether the picture you have is real or imagined.

Start with real people and objects, e.g., "Your Mum, she's a real person"; "a bus is a real vehicle". Then add a fantasy character, e.g., a wizard, and explain why he is a fantasy character, he has magic powers and only happens in stories, he's not real, etc.

Repeat for the rest of the fantasy/reality pictures, explaining the difference as you go.

Sort the words for real and imaginary into the two piles and ask the child which words he knows.

Add some words and pictures to the Friendship book on a page headed, 'Fantasy and Reality'.

Explain that sometimes people might tell stories with imagined characters in them, and we have to listen carefully to hear whether the story is real or imaginary.

Read out one of the scripts from the Resource.

Ask the child to decide if the story belongs in the fantasy pile or in the reality pile and discuss the clues in the story that made it real or make-believe. Repeat for the rest of the scripts.

Now read a mixed script by combining elements of events, characters, and objects from the scripts in the Resource, e.g., start with a real script then change halfway through to introduce a fantasy element to see if the child can identify the change in content.

Ask the child to change the script to make it a real/believable story.

Repeat with a few scripts until the child is confidently identifying the fantasy elements and replacing these with good suggestions for real events, characters, and objects.

Add one script for fantasy and one for reality into his Friendship book and label. If the child can read, use a written version of the scripts and read together to identify the different words that indicate fantasy and reality. Cross out fantasy words and change them to real things.

Personalisation

After a few stories, add the child's particular fantasy interest to some of the scripts and support him to remove the fantasy elements from the script as before.

Ask if he ever talks about stories when he is talking to people at home or in school. Discuss that this might be confusing as people will think he is talking about real events, people, or objects.

Discuss how to make it better, e.g., by only talking about real things, explaining that you are talking about a game or story you have made up. Add a summary to the child's Friendship book.

SCIP Phase 2: SUSI 5
Resource

SUSI 5.2 Understanding the impact of preferred interests
Activity 4 Resource: Understanding fantasy and reality

Write the following words on separate cards. Use plain script and black ink for the real words and multi-coloured inks and cursive scripts for the fantasy words as an extra cue if needed.

Real words: Real, everyday, usual, normal, ordinary, believable, true, possible, convincing, true to life, factual, correct, accurate.

Fantasy words: Daydream, imagination, pretending, make-believe, fantasy, made up, unrealistic, impossible, fictional, imaginary.

Real images: Any images of real items and well-known people the child will recognise.

Fantasy images: Magic wand, Tardis, sonic screwdriver, spectotronic liquid, time machine, talking animals, fairy dust, shrinking potion, singing plants, dragons, Harry Potter, fairy godmother, witch, Homer Simpson.

Sample scripts can be combined to produce a mixed story.

Real scripts

❖ I am in the park. It is a sunny day. I am sitting on the grass with my friends. We are eating sandwiches and crisps. Mason has brought his football so we can play after lunch

❖ the pilot has told us to fasten our seatbelts. The aeroplane has just taken off. The houses and people on the ground look smaller and smaller as the plane climbs higher into the sky

❖ some children are making a model of a castle. Other children are finding out about castles using the Internet. I am looking in the book corner for a book on the history of castles

❖ there are lots of different animals here. I have been to see the monkeys and the giraffe. There is a noise – it is a lion roaring. After lunch we are going to see the penguins being fed

❖ I went to see the new Batman film. It was so amazing. He has a car that flies and spins around in the air. I think they used loads of special effects

Fantasy scripts

❖ I am sitting on a broomstick, flying up above the treetops. I look down and wave to my Mum and Dad

❖ we are on a mission to travel to the centre of the earth. We have an enormous digger and a special vehicle that can withstand extremely high temperatures

❖ people are shouting and cheering. I am wearing shiny armour and riding a horse. I have gone back in time to be a knight

❖ there is an animal that can breathe fire. Everyone is very scared. The animal opens a huge pair of wings and flies into the sky. It is a dragon!

❖ yesterday, instead of going to school, I went back in time to the time of the dinosaurs. I saw a Tyrannosaurus Rex. It was so cool. I came back home and drew a picture of it

SCIP Phase 2: SUSI 5

SUSI 5.2 Understanding the impact of preferred interests

Activity 5: The impact of fantasy worlds

Purpose and target

To help the child to understand the impact of fantasy worlds on learning and friendship.

Materials

Child's Friendship book from Activity 1: This activity forms one part of making a Friendship book for use throughout Phase 2.

Three puppets or three laminated figures; two children and one adult.

Emotions ladders and Book of Feelings from SUSI 2 work.

Procedure

Introduce the first character, "This is my friend Daisy Daydreamer. Daisy loves to watch TV. Her favourite cartoon is Scooby Doo. When Daisy Daydreamer isn't watching TV, she likes to think about Scooby Doo and remember what happens in the show. This is called daydreaming".

Act out Daisy talking about the latest cartoon of Scooby Doo or equivalent.

Explain that although Daisy likes to think about Scooby Doo, sometimes it gets her into trouble.

Introduce the adult character as a teacher who asks Daisy a question, e.g., to count to 20.

Daisy starts off well, "1, 2, 3, 4, 5", but then says, "Oh no, we should run away, there's a ghost coming. Quick, we need to hide!".

Explain that this means that Daisy has drifted off into a Scooby Doo daydream.

The teacher is confused and she says, "Daisy you need to think about your work. You might have to stay in at playtime to do your work".

Discuss what happened. Why did Daisy start talking about Scooby Doo?

Discuss the teacher's feelings. How does Daisy feel now? Why shouldn't Daisy daydream about Scooby Doo in lessons? Refer to the child's emotions ladders to show changes in feeling from OK to upset for Daisy and explain why talking about Scooby Doo is not a good idea.

Repeat but this time set up a role-play showing Daisy playing with a friend in the playground. Daisy starts the game well and they are having fun but then she starts to talk about Scooby Doo again and wants to act out events from the cartoons that don't fit the game.

Stop and ask the child what is happening. Ask him to give advice to Daisy on how to stay in the game, ask to play a Scooby Doo game after this one, etc.

Meta-challenge

Continue to act this out until her friends leave her out of the game because they don't want to think about Scooby Doo.

Discuss how everyone feels. Refer to the child's emotions ladders to show the change from happy and playing to lonely and sad.

Agree solutions so that Daisy can think about her favourite thing at a different time, but that when she is with her friends she can think about the games and listen to her friends.

Personalisation

Use the child's particular fantasy interest and language to present a situation that he might encounter. As far as the child will accept, discuss changes and options to improve interactions.

Write a summary sketch or story in the child's Friendship book.

SCIP Phase 2: SUSI 5

SUSI 5.3 Understanding friendship skills

Activity 1: Friendship role-play

Purpose and target

To enable the child to practise different friendship skills, consolidate understanding of interests in friendship, and to practice friendship role-plays.

Materials

Child's Friendship book from Activity 1: This activity forms one part of making a Friendship book for use throughout Phase 2.

Composite pictures of children in different settings, e.g., playing tennis, football, walking to the park, skipping together, running around, junk modelling, construction toys.

Select pictures that do **not** show any challenges in the interaction.

Procedure

Lay out the first picture and say, "We are going to pretend to be the children in these pictures. I will be him and you can be the other boy".

Start a role-play to demonstrate: Talking about the project they are doing, giving compliments to the other person, asking for equipment, for a turn, to help with something.

After the role-play, stop and talk about the things that have been said in the role-play and write these down in the child's Friendship book on a new page headed, 'Talking with my friends'.

Against each comment or question draw feeling faces to indicate OK and happy reactions to the questions and comments.

Repeat with a new scenario and demonstrate a similar range of questions, comments, and compliments in the play.

Role-reversal

Encourage the child to take a number of different roles and to develop insight into what different characters might do, what they might be thinking, how they might feel, and the language they might use.

Make sure the child can demonstrate all the skills that have been role-played.

Meta-challenge

When the child can act out a few roles and ask questions or make matching comments, introduce a meta-challenge by not answering or not asking any questions in return. Stop and discuss the impact on the interaction and what the other character will think and feel, e.g., he is ignoring me, he doesn't want to play with me, etc.

Write a summary sketch or story in the child's Friendship book.

SCIP Phase 2: SUSI 5

SUSI 5.3 Understanding friendship skills

Activity 2: Identifying and solving problems in friendship

Purpose and target

To enable the child to identify a range of different friendship problems and learn how to resolve issues such as sharing, accidents, and being left out.

Materials

Child's Friendship book from Activity 1: This activity forms one part of making a Friendship book for use throughout Phase 2.

Pictures that show an upset or problem in the interaction between children, e.g., Black Sheep Press Talkabout School and Talkabout Friends series, or draw scenarios to show, e.g., playing a computer game with one child looking bored, one child on a bike while the other watches, and one child falling on top of another at the bottom of a slide.

Procedure

Add 'Solving problems in friendships' as a heading on a new page in the child's Friendship book. Explain that this work is to solve problems in friendships. Lay out the first picture and explain that sometimes things go wrong with friends, and we need to be able to work out what is going wrong and work out what to do to fix it.

Look at the first picture and talk about the problem, support the child to identify what has happened and understand why. Refer to strategies in SUSI 1 to support this.

Write the problem and the reasons in the child's Friendship book, e.g., sometimes when the children are playing their computer game, one person takes too long, and the other person gets bored/cross about it. Explain possible reasons why, e.g., one player is better than the other and takes a longer turn.

Introduce the idea of three possible endings, a 'sad ending' where the situation ends badly for all; a 'good ending' where they come up with a solution so that everyone is happy, and an 'OK ending'. An OK ending is one where things are OK for everyone, e.g., change to a different game. OK endings also include a solution for 'next time', e.g., spend time practising the game alone so that 'next time' they will be more evenly matched.

Write or draw all three endings and add speech and thinking bubbles to indicate what is happening. Use key phrases and colour coding to indicate different outcomes, e.g., blue for OK, green for good.

Start a role-play to demonstrate the sad, OK, and happy endings. Say, "Let's start by making things even worse and making a sad ending. This boy is going to snatch the computer console away from his friend".

Discuss each ending as you act out different choices the child can make and make notes in the child's Friendship book on what can go wrong and how to sort out problems. Record useful words to use and how to ask for help.

Repeat with at least three more scenarios and engage the child in identifying and solving the problems. Encourage use of mediating language and emphasise the alternative outcomes.

Meta-challenge

In role-play, ignore the child's attempts to solve the problem and reach a point where help is needed from an adult or walk away from the game.

SCIP Phase 2: SUSI 5

SUSI 5.3 Understanding friendship skills
Activity 3: Identifying and solving problems in friendship (personalised)

Purpose and target

To enable the child to identify a range of different friendship problems and identify issues that occur in his own friendships.

Materials

Child's Friendship book from Activity 1: This activity forms one part of making a Friendship book for use throughout Phase 2.

A list of recent upsets experienced by the child in friendships from the child's ISCP or by report from staff and parents.

This activity needs to be sensitively managed, preferably when a strong alliance has been established and the child is robust enough to cope with direct feedback.

Procedure

Following from Activity 2, remind the child that sometimes we have problems with our friends, and we need to work out how to make things OK for everyone if we can.

Explain that this work is to think about ways to help you get it right with your friends.

Start to draw a picture and say, "This is you at playtime in school". Add a friend and say, "Here's your friend Jack. I know that sometimes when you play with Jack, you get upset and he gets upset too. Here you are, you are both looking sad. Oh no, what can have happened?". Use this picture as the sad ending for the story.

Start to draw a sequence of pictures (as in LP2.2) from the beginning of the reported upset and use the actual events, words used, and names of people involved.

Repeat the steps in Activity 2 by working through the story to the point of upset, explaining all the reasons and thoughts and feelings.

Encourage the child to contribute, ask for his thoughts and feelings and get him to draw and write on the picture sequence or post it notes. Call this the sad ending.

Now tell the story again, but this time stop before the point of upset and insert a few blank cards to the story. Support the child to come up with ideas to make this an OK or happy ending. These may have been suggested to you by parents and teachers.

Use a different colour pen to indicate the alternative actions and words that can be helpful to reach a different ending, e.g., original story in black ink, OK ending in blue, and happy ending in green.

Refer back to similar upsets from Activity 2.

Emphasise that happy endings may be unrealistic and that OK endings are usually easy to think of.

Write up key words and solutions for one or two scenarios in the child's Friendships book and consider whether this is a suitable Phase 3 target.

Note any misunderstandings, over-reactions, and inflexibility to minor upsets and revise teaching using SUSI 1, SUSI 2, and SUSI 3 activities as needed to support friendship skills. If the child needs support to take others' perspectives into account, revise SUSI 4 activities.

SCIP Phase 2: SUSI 5

SUSI 5.3 Understanding friendship skills
Activity 4: Understanding friendship (personalised)

Purpose and target

To provide an opportunity for the child to reflect on his own friendships and what he wants in a friend. To demonstrate an understanding of shared interests and qualities that make a good friend.

Materials

Large sheet of blank paper and coloured pens.

Procedure

Tell the child that the task is to produce a poster describing his ideal friend.

The child should draw the friend in the centre and label the picture with the qualities and features which make a good friend.

Support him to remember the work that has been completed on interests and to think about people he is friends with or things he has observed children in his class doing.

Discuss qualities that make a good friend, e.g., kind, sharing toys, taking turns, etc.

Use the first letters of the word 'friend' to come up with a list of interests and qualities. Take each letter in turn and add a word or phrase that describes an aspect of friendship, e.g., F for fun, R for remembering what they like to do, I for inviting them to your house, E for eating together, N for noticing how they feel, and D for doing things you both like.

Discuss and prompt as necessary, using other words for friendship to decorate the poster.

Invite the child to add drawings of their interests and write names of their friends on the poster.

You can divide the poster into interests at the top and qualities at the bottom to help the child conceptualise these ideas.

Observe what aspects of understanding friendship and interests the child has learned and what needs further development.

PRAG CONTENT TABLES AND INTERVENTION ACTIVITIES

Pragmatics (PRAG) Content table

Pragmatics (PRAG)

Sections	Objectives			
PRAG 1 **Turn-taking and reciprocity**	PRAG 1.1 Understanding how to take turns	PRAG 1.2 Understanding verbal turn-taking	PRAG 1.3 Consolidating turn-taking skills	
PRAG 2 **Conversation and metapragmatic skills**	PRAG 2.1 Enhanced listening skills	PRAG 2.2 Understanding speaker roles	PRAG 2.3 Giving information	PRAG 2.4 Developing metapragmatic awareness
PRAG 3 **Understanding information requirements**	PRAG 3.1 Understanding impact of missing information	PRAG 3.2 Understanding impact of too much information	PRAG 3.3 Understanding matching context and talk	PRAG 3.4 Understanding information requirements in personal conversation
PRAG 4 **Understanding and managing topic in conversation**	PRAG 4.1 Identifying topics	PRAG 4.2 Understanding topic change conventions	PRAG 4.3 Consolidating topic skills	
PRAG **5 Understanding and improving discourse style**	PRAG 5.1 Understanding different styles in interaction	PRAG 5.2 Understanding and using conventions of interaction style	PRAG 5.3 Consolidating interaction style	

DOI: 10.4324/9781032706641-5

PRAG 1 Intervention content table

SCIP Phase 2	PRAG 1 Intervention content table

PRAG 1 Turn-taking and reciprocity

PRAG 1 Information

PRAG 1.1 Understanding how to take turns

1 Understanding the rules of turn-taking (non-verbal)

2 Understanding the rules of turn-taking (verbal)

PRAG 1.2 Understanding verbal turn-taking

1 Understanding the sequence of initiation and response

2 Modifying the sequence of initiation and response

3 Enhancing reciprocity in conversation

4 Understanding turn-taking in conversation (simple)

5 Understanding turn-taking in conversation (complex)

PRAG 1.3 Consolidating turn-taking skills

1 Enhancing turn-taking skills in conversation

2 Enhancing turn-taking skills in conversation (personalised)

SCIP Phase 2: PRAG 1

Information

PRAG 1 Turn-taking and reciprocity

The purpose of this Section is to help your child understand the rules of turn-taking in conversation and to be able to take turns in a reciprocal conversation. The Section starts by teaching rules for turn-taking in games.

These rules are:

- ❖ decide who will go first
- ❖ wait for the other person to finish
- ❖ when it's your turn, don't wait – get going!
- ❖ let everyone have a turn in order

The words he will learn are: first, next, last, my turn, your turn, before, after, wait, fair, not fair. Visual representations for turn-taking rules will be used to help your child understand and discuss them. Once these rules and words are established, your child will practise taking turns in conversation and will learn how these rules, and a few new rules apply to conversation:

- ❖ pay attention/look at the other person/watch them to see if they have finished
- ❖ listen carefully/think about the words
- ❖ try not to interrupt

Through role-play and using puppets to show rules and rule breaks, your child will understand the impact of using and not using turn-taking rules in conversation. Turn-taking in conversation (reciprocity) relies on being aware of subtle signs that the speaker has finished talking. When he has understood the basic rules of turn-taking, your child will learn how to look out for and interpret subtle turn-taking cues in conversation such as, when the speaker has finished his answer, he may look up at the other person expectantly, and the pitch of his voice goes up or changes.

An understanding of the consequences of not taking turns in conversation will be taught. Links between people's feelings and not taking turns will be covered, e.g., bored, confused, and irritated. Your child will understand the impact of not giving the other person a turn in conversation, or of not taking a turn. Work in this Section builds towards your child being able to reflect on his/her own turn-taking skills. The focus is on developing awareness of these skills and the impact their use and non-use has on the interaction. Specific words and phrases will be taught to help your child talk about his/her own conversation skills.

Recent actual conversations with your child will be used to help him reflect on what has been done well and what he needs to practise.

How you can help

Teaching in this Section will be tailored to meet your child's needs. Please provide information from your child's recent actual experiences on how he typically performs in conversation. Please provide information on the words that your child will be familiar with for talking about taking turns in conversation, e.g., "I asked you a question, now it's your turn to talk", etc.

SCIP Phase 2: PRAG 1

PRAG 1.1 Understanding how to take turns

Activity 1: Understanding the rules of turn-taking (non-verbal)

Purpose and target

To help the child to understand basic turn-taking rules and vocabulary in a game.

Materials

Board or card games with opportunity for many turns, e.g., Snail's Pace Race.
Set of turn-taking rules and vocabulary written on blank cards:

- ❖ decide who will go first
- ❖ wait for the other person to finish
- ❖ watch them to see if they have finished
- ❖ when it's your turn, don't wait – get going!
- ❖ don't interrupt
- ❖ finish your turn as quick as you can
- ❖ let everyone have a turn in order

Vocabulary: First, next, last, my turn, your turn, before, after, wait, fair, not fair.

Procedure

Explain that playing the chosen game helps us to practise taking turns. Talk through each of the turn-taking rules and set them out on the table.

Decide who will go first and point to this card. Let the child start, wait for him to finish, and then point to that card. Say, "We agreed you could start, so you had a turn and now it's my turn".

Carry on playing the game and talk about each rule explicitly as you go.

Repeat the rules and vocabulary related to each player's actions throughout.

Meta-challenge

Play another game and, as you play, break one rule at a time. Explain that this time you want to find out what happens when the rules are broken.

Start the game by agreeing who will start and then do the opposite. Stop and talk about what happened: "How did you feel when I grabbed the dice? Was that fair?".

Get the game going and break another rule and talk about it in the same way to demonstrate the consequences of each rule break.

Help the child to write or stick the rules in his workbook.

Role-reversal meta-challenge

Play a new game and ask the child to deliberately break one of the rules for you to identify which rule has been broken. Continue with a few rule breaks and discuss the child's experience of rule breaks when playing with others. Note examples in his ISCP for future work if needed.

SCIP Phase 2: PRAG 1

PRAG 1.1 Understanding how to take turns

Activity 2: Understanding the rules of turn-taking (verbal)

Purpose and target

To help the child to understand basic turn-taking rules and vocabulary in a structured verbal interaction.

Materials

Picture sequence sets, e.g., from Schubi Tell Me About It.

Non-verbal turn-taking cards from PRAG 3.1.1.

Verbal turn-taking rule cards:

- ❖ pay attention/look at the other person/watch them to see if they have finished
- ❖ listen carefully/think about the words
- ❖ don't interrupt

Vocabulary: First, next, last, my turn, your turn, before, after, wait, interrupt

Procedure

Remind the child that the rules are the same as those practised in Activity 1 with only three new rules to remember. Talk through each of the turn-taking rules and set them out on the table and explain that now we are practising taking turns to talk.

Set out the story sequence in order and agree that you will go first, point to this rule.

Start the story off by talking about the first picture. Stop and talk about what rules the child was following: Looking, listening carefully, waiting for you to finish.

Ask the child to take the next turn and again reflect on the rules used: Stop when you have finished.

Repeat with at least three new stories to talk about the other rules.

Meta-challenge

Repeat with another story but this time break one rule at a time. Explain that this time you want to find out what happens when the rules are broken.

Start the story after agreeing who will start and then do the opposite. Stop and talk about what happened: "How did you feel when I interrupted/didn't start my turn? What should I do instead?".

Break another rule and talk about it in the same way to demonstrate the consequences of each rule break.

Help the child to write or stick the rules for taking turns when talking in his workbook.

Role-reversal meta-challenge

Start another story and ask the child to break the rules and for you to identify what rule has been broken. Continue with a few rule breaks and discuss the child's experience of rule breaks when talking with others. Note examples in his ISCP for future work in PRAG 1.3.

SCIP Phase 2: PRAG 1

PRAG 1.2 Understanding verbal turn-taking

Activity 1: Understanding the sequence of initiation and response

Purpose and target

To help the child to understand the sequences of listener and speaker talk and develop metapragmatic awareness of reciprocity in conversation.

Materials

Pictures of familiar social situations, e.g., from Schubi Tell Me About It sequencing cards or Colorcards: Daily Living Skills: Social Behaviour.

Speech bubble sticky notes and different coloured pens for each speaker.

Prepared simple conversation sequences with each speaker's initiations and responses written on a separate speech bubble for a few of the social situations.

Procedure

Start with one scene and explain that you are going to think about what each person says to start the conversation and keep it going.

Start with the first person and write his/her words on a speech bubble sticky note.

Write what the other person says in response and stick both to a blank page and draw an arrow between them to show the order of initiations and responses.

Repeat with another comment from the first speaker and another reply.

Repeat, drawing arrows to show how one utterance is linked to the next and discuss that these words go together because they make sense together.

Move two replies to different initiations and explain that these don't make sense now. Emphasise that the things people say to each other should make sense.

Repeat with new scenes and new conversation starters. Ask the child to contribute follow up comments and questions to keep the conversation going.

As you work, aim for a set of different directional conversations, e.g., showing that both people can initiate and respond, both can ask questions, etc.

Role-play

Role-play the scene taking a character each and using the scripts as a prompt, but try to extend the turns with new contributions from you and the child as it builds. Observe the child's performance in this and make a note of conversational strengths and needs on his ISCP.

SCIP Phase 2: PRAG 1

PRAG 1.2 Understanding verbal turn-taking

Activity 2: Modifying the sequence of initiation and response

Purpose and target

To enable the child to modify a sequence of listener and speaker talk by paying attention to the meaning of each utterance and to facilitate metapragmatic awareness of reciprocity in conversation.

Materials

Several conversation sequences prepared in Activity 1 with each speaker's initiations and responses written on a speech bubble sticky note and the arrows showing the direction of talk.

Procedure

Following from Activity 1, set out one complete conversation and revise that it all fits together because the conversation makes sense.

Meta-challenge

Explain that you are going to mix the conversation up so that it doesn't make sense. Ask the child to cover his eyes while you mix it up by moving one speech bubble only.

Ask him to read through the conversation and find the speech bubble you moved.

Discuss what happened to the conversation when the order was mixed up, e.g., it is confusing.

Ask the child to reset the conversation and explain you are going to make other changes for him to work out. Each time ask the child to cover his eyes while you make a change.

Repeat to demonstrate other reciprocity mix-ups as follows:

❖ questions in place of answers so that a series of questions is presented
❖ add a blank speech bubble in place of a response to indicate no response
❖ add all the comments together after one question

Each time, discuss the impact of the mix-ups and what happens when we don't follow the rules to keep the conversation going, e.g., the speaker might feel confused, the listener doesn't know what to say, or wasn't listening, etc. Explain, e.g., that each question needs a reply and if the listener is confused, he can ask the other person to repeat what they said or explain it more clearly.

Role-reversal

Engage in role-reversal and ask the child to have a go at breaking up the conversation for you to detect. As you find the change he made, discuss to reinforce metapragmatic understanding.

SCIP Phase 2: PRAG 1

PRAG 1.2 Understanding verbal turn-taking

Activity 3: Enhancing reciprocity in conversation

Purpose and target

To help the child to develop metapragmatic awareness of how he manages reciprocity in conversation and be able to signal this awareness in his own conversations.

Materials

A sheet of paper with two columns of blank speech bubbles.
Speech bubble sticky notes.

Procedure

Following from Activity 2, explain that this task is to think about conversations that really happen.

Start a short conversation with the child and when it ends explain that you are going to write down what was said.

Write the main points of the conversation into the speech bubbles as it happened.

Start at the beginning and point out the initiations and responses as in Activity 1. Draw arrows to show the order of initiations and responses.

Engage the child in reflecting on the conversation to find what went well and discuss turn-taking skills used and add any new skills as needed to reflect the chat, e.g., "you answered my question".

Repeat with at least one more conversation with no interruptions to establish the child in monitoring the skills used.

Meta-challenge

Start another conversation and provoke an a meta-challenge in comprehension by being vague or using words the child will not know.

Write it out as before, exactly as it happened.

When you reach the meta-challenge, e.g., no response or no request for clarification, pause and discuss with the child what happened. Explain that if he is confused, he can ask the other person to repeat what they said or explain it.

Repeat and ask several questions in a row without pause for the answers. Write it down showing that only one person was speaking and discuss how this feels for the other person and what they can do instead. Refer to the turn-taking rules from PRAG 1.1 as needed.

Personalisation

Start another conversation and act out one of the child's reciprocity behaviours and write it down.

Discuss how this feels for the other person, and whether a change should be made. Label what happened, e.g., too many questions here.

Write down a potential self-help strategy or revision to the interchange and place this on the sticky note sequence.

Engage the child in a repeat of the same conversation with the repaired phrase added.

Observe the child's level of awareness of this and whether he can show self-awareness to the point of adopting the self-help strategy.

SCIP Phase 2: PRAG 1

PRAG 1.2 Understanding verbal turn-taking

Activity 4: Understanding turn-taking in conversation (simple)

Purpose and target

To help the child understand the impact of using and not using turn-taking rules in conversation.

Materials

Pictures for conversation topics, e.g., Schubi Combimage cards.

Two puppets, e.g., Rabbit and Sheep.

Non-verbal and verbal turn-taking cards and vocabulary from PRAG 1.1 activities.

Procedure

Write or show the turn-taking rules to remind the child of these and say, "Now we are practising taking turns in conversation". Explain that the puppets are friends, and they are going to have a chat about something they both like. Use a Combimage card to represent the topic. Ask the child to watch the puppets and see what rules they know.

Get the conversation going between the puppets and choose one rule to focus on to model turn-taking. Point out successful use of turn-taking rules by the puppets.

Repeat using two or three different topics to cover all rules previously taught.

In each conversation, stop to point out the skills used, either immediately, or at the end of the chat.

Meta-challenge

Start a new conversation between the puppets and break one rule. Observe the child's response and support him to comment on the rule break and agree an alternative. Give prompts, if necessary, e.g., "Rabbit didn't start to speak when it was his turn. Sheep could say, 'Hey Rabbit, I asked you a question, but you didn't answer. Shall I ask you again?'".

Include speaker role features (talking at the same time, not agreeing who will start, talking for too long) and in listener role (taking too long to reply, interrupting when it is not his turn).

Make a note of the rules, feelings, and solutions in the child's workbook.

Role-reversal meta-challenge

Select a new topic and ask the child to control one puppet and break the rules for you to identify what rule has been broken.

Personalisation

Use the child's usual turn-taking behaviour and discuss what happened, why, and whether it could be changed. Observe the child's level of awareness of this and whether he can give any self-help strategies.

SCIP Phase 2: PRAG 1

PRAG 1.2 Understanding verbal turn-taking

Activity 5: Understanding turn-taking in conversation (complex)

Purpose and target

To enhance the child's understanding of subtle turn-taking cues in conversation.

Materials

Pictures for conversation topics (Schubi Combimage cards).

Two puppets, e.g., Rabbit and Sheep.

Subtle turn-taking cues on cards: speaker stops speaking/has finished their answer; looks up at the other person expectantly; pitch of voice goes up.

Procedure

Following from Activity 4, remind the child about the turn-taking rules and say, "Now we are practising listening and watching the speaker closely to 'work out' when it is time to take a turn". Talk about each cue and explain that the puppets are going to show us each one in turn. Use a topic card and ask the child to pay attention to the puppet who is speaking very closely. This activity is delivered slowly, and each turn is discussed in detail, pointing out the cues and rules both puppets are using.

Get the conversation going between the puppets and choose one cue to focus on. Explain that Rabbit knows it is his turn to speak because Sheep *has finished talking*. Now Rabbit needs to *get going* with his reply (rule). When Rabbit finishes, he will look up at Sheep. Explain that now Sheep knows it is his turn because Rabbit *has finished talking* and he *is looking at* Sheep. Now Sheep will talk and will use *a rising intonation* to indicate that he wants Rabbit to comment or answer a question.

Talk about the way the voice sounds different. Repeat the comment with and without the intonation change to make sure the child has picked up on this. Repeat with at least five topics. Write the conversation down if this helps.

Write the cues and how the listener should respond in the child's workbook.

SCIP Phase 2: PRAG 1

PRAG 1.3 Consolidating turn-taking skills

Activity 1: Enhancing turn-taking skills in conversation

Purpose and target

To help the child in consolidating turn-taking skills for conversation.

Materials

Verbal and non-verbal turn-taking rule cards from previous work in this Section.

Up to three new puppets/characters not used in this section before (to act as not knowing the rules).

Set of simple questions to ask with a tick box next to each, e.g., "How old are you?", "Do you have brothers and sisters?".

Procedure

Remind the child about the turn-taking rules and cues and say, "Now we are practising listening and watching the new speakers closely to see whether they can take turns". Explain that the game is to find out some things about the new puppets by asking questions and listening to the answers. Show the child the list of questions and ask him to tick the question when the puppet answers it. Do not tell the child to expect rule breaks. This activity should be fun and relaxed. If the child is confused, go back and repeat PRAG 1.2 activities or make it explicit that the puppet has not learned the rules.

Get the first puppet ready and support the child to ask the first question. The puppet will break all the rules of turn-taking. Stop after each question and ask the child to identify which rule of turn-taking has been broken and discuss how that makes him feel. What should the puppet have done instead?

Write down the rule break on a separate card in a different colour (red), e.g., not answering the right question.

Repeat for all rules and cues and discuss with the child.

If the child reports his experience of conversation rule breaks, make a note and explain that this will be covered in Activity 2 and move to Activity 2.

If the child needs support to identify any rule breaks focus in on that rule break, repeat with a new puppet and new conversation.

Role-reversal meta-challenge

Now ask the child to act for another new puppet and explain that this puppet doesn't know
    anything about turn-taking and so it will break some rules. Select a new topic and ask
    the child to break the rules for you to identify what rule has been broken.

Talk about how the rule breaks make you feel (bored, confused, irritated).

Draw a picture of the new puppets in the workbook and write down the mistakes they made.

Add a sketch summary of this to the child's Book of Feelings from SUSI 2 work if useful.

SCIP Phase 2: PRAG 1

PRAG 1.3 Consolidating turn-taking skills

Activity 2: Enhancing turn-taking skills in conversation (personalised)

Purpose and target

To help the child to understand his own turn-taking skills and to consolidate turn-taking skills for conversation.

Materials

Verbal and non-verbal turn-taking rule cards from previous work in this Section.

Pictures for general conversation topics (Schubi Combimage cards).

Pictures for conversation topics based on personal interests and recent conversations reported as having problems with turn-taking.

Examples of recent and recurrent examples of turn-taking from the child's ISCP.

Procedure

Remind the child about the turn-taking rules and cues and say, "Now we are practising listening and watching each other in a conversation about things we like". Do not tell the child to expect rule breaks. This activity should be fun and as close to a natural conversation as possible. Get the first conversation going on a general topic and stop as soon as an example of good turn-taking has occurred. Point this out and talk about the rule the child used and how that makes you feel. Continue the conversation in this way, talking and stopping to comment on the rules as they are observed.

If there is a turn-taking clash, pause to see if he can use a self-help strategy. If not, stop the interaction and say, "Something got a bit stuck there. I feel confused/bored, etc." Ask, "What went wrong? Do you know?" Discuss with the child and point out what they did and how that made you feel (bored, confused, irritated). Talk about how these feelings relate to the rule breaks as in Activity 1.

Repeat with general and personal topics as the child shows awareness and ability to comment on his own turn-taking skills.

Use a topic that has been reported by parents or teachers to be challenging and observe the child's turn-taking skills in this topic.

Draw a picture of the child talking to the practitioner in his workbook and write down the skills the child can use easily. Add a smiley face next to these rules. Make a list of things the child needs to remember and draw an OK face next to these. Explain that these are the skills he can get better at.

PRAG 2 Intervention content table

SCIP Phase 2	PRAG 2 Intervention content table

PRAG 2 Conversation and metapragmatic skills

PRAG 2 Information

PRAG 2.1 Enhanced listening skills

1 Understanding listening skills

2 Understanding looking in listening

PRAG 2.2 Understanding speaker roles

1 Asking wh– questions

2 Asking yes/no questions

3 Understanding useful questions plus Resource

4 Understanding multiple questions

PRAG 2.3 Giving information

1 Giving clear messages

2 Responding to requests for further information

PRAG 2.4 Developing metapragmatic awareness

1 Metapragmatic awareness of conversation conventions

2 Metapragmatic awareness of conversation conventions (personalised)

SCIP Phase 2: PRAG 2

Information

PRAG 2 Conversation and metapragmatic skills

The purpose of this Section is to help your child understand rules for successful conversation, such as asking questions that match the context, giving information clearly, and checking for and modifying misunderstandings. The focus is on developing awareness of these skills and the impact their use and non-use has on the interaction. Specific words and phrases will be taught to help your child talk about and think about his/her own conversation skills.

Work in this Section develops your child's understanding of a range of different skills required in conversation and is intended to guide the practitioner to a better understanding of your child's strengths and needs in conversation management. Children with persistent social communication needs can sometimes know a conversation rule while still struggling to use that rule. Work in this Section will provide information on your child's knowledge of conversation management, his/her ability to use conversation skills for mutual reward, and insight into what he needs to do to enhance conversational ability. This Section has a specific focus on developing a range of strategies to help with active listening. Targets for conversation management will be derived from work completed in this Section and added into the child's plan for intervention.

Photographs, drawings, and other visual representations for conversation rules will be used to help your child understand and discuss them. Your child will be taught specific vocabulary for conversation skills and will learn about the impact on feelings at a simple level of not using a skill. A chart of listening skills, created in Phase 1, will be used to help focus his attention on what he is doing well that helps listening and which skills are needed to be a better listener.

Recent actual conversations with the child will be used to help him reflect on what he does well and what he needs to practise.

How you can help

Teaching in this Section will be tailored to meet your child's needs. Please provide information from your child's recent actual experiences on how he typically performs in conversation and what skills you consider a priority for intervention. Please provide information on the words that your child will be familiar with for talking about conversation.

You can help by using your child's listening skills chart in class and by using the same words and phrases to talk to your child about listening skills, e.g., look at the person speaking, or ask for help if you are stuck. Use the chart to remind your child which specific behaviours have been achieved and which ones he needs to practise. Use incentives such as drawing smiles under each skill as they are noticed, by starting a smile when you notice a skill that needs to be used and encourage your child to try to gain the complete smile by, e.g., saying, "I think you can get that smile if you listen to the questions". The listening skills chart should be phased out over time. Liaise with your practitioner to agree which skills can be removed from the chart and how the skills can be practised without the chart. Your child may be able to draw his own version from memory, showing what he can remember.

SCIP Phase 2: PRAG 2

PRAG 2.1 Enhanced listening skills

Activity 1: Understanding listening skills

Purpose and target

To reinforce the child's metapragmatic awareness of his own listening skills and support him to become able to self-monitor.

Materials

Chart of listening skills chart created in Phase 1 MPA activities. The chart should contain skills, such as thinking about the words, looking at the speaker, knowing what was said, asking for help.

Short extracts from age-appropriate texts.

Procedure

Discuss with the child each listening skill on his chart and amend it by adding any other skills the child can now begin to practise; remove any the child has mastered.

Explain that the task is to use each of the skills on the chart while listening to a short story.

Explain that the child will be asked to reflect on his own listening skills at the end of the story.

Select one skill to practise first. Read a short extract from the story and stop to give feedback on the selected skill. Ask the child how he did. Guide him to an accurate report of how he performed before you start reading again.

Instruct the child to select a different listening skill and reflect at the end on how he performed.

Repeat with all skills and reflect at the end of the story on which skills were achieved and those that need practice.

Use a suitable means of rewarding the use of specific skills, e.g., smiley faces, and use an incentive to practise the challenging ones, e.g., double smiles for trying not to fidget, small smiles for effort.

Repeat with a new story and explain that this time you want the child to use as many of the skills as possible while you read.

Stop and support the child to reflect on the skills he used as before. Aim for accurate reflection.

Reinforce that the child can think about whether he is listening or not, and if he is not listening, he can help himself to listen by using the skills on the chart.

Ask the child which skills can be improved and which are easy to do. Discuss how the chart can help keep track of listening skills and explain that it will be used in all activities from now on.

At the end, the child will have a chart of listening skills that need consolidation. Copy this chart for home and school and keep a copy in the child's file.

SCIP Phase 2: PRAG 2

PRAG 2.1 Enhanced listening skills
Activity 2: Understanding looking in listening
Purpose and target

To reinforce the child's metapragmatic awareness of the role of looking when listening to a speaker and understand the consequences of not looking.

Materials

Puppets and small toys to hide inside one of the puppets.
I know/I don't know cards from Phase 1 CM activities if needed.
Emotions ladders from work in SUSI 2.

Procedure

Introduce the task: "Today we're going to talk about the ways in which people look at each other when they are talking. Sometimes we look at faces and sometimes we look around".

Ask the child to draw a picture of someone with big eyes to represent looking. Discuss different ways of looking at the other person and name them, e.g., staring, "I'm staring at you now – staring means looking at you for a long time without looking away".

Repeat to model 'looking away' and 'looking to listen'.

Use two puppets to model staring, looking away, and looking to listen in a short exchange.

Explain the role of looking in conversation – to pick up on emotions, showing that you are listening, and showing that you are interested.

Using both puppets, start a conversation and make one look away. Have the second puppet hide a small object.

The first puppet then asks where the toy is. Discuss why the first puppet doesn't know where it is, because he didn't look at the other puppet. Use the 'I don't know' cards and the child's listening chart from Phase 1 if useful.

Repeat with child watching the puppets closely and emphasise why he knows which toy was hidden, and say, e.g., "You know because you were looking".

Discuss the emotions that might arise when someone stares/looks away/has a cross face/ has a big smile. Use emotion vocabulary the child knows and refer to emotions ladders from work in SUSI 2 if useful.

Role-reversal

Ask the child to control one of the puppets to show looking while listening. Observe whether the child is looking to listen while controlling the puppet and discuss how the puppet helped or didn't help.

Personalisation

Repeat with the child in conversation with a puppet and have the puppet walk away or hide under the desk when the child looks away.

Discuss what happened: "Why did the puppet hide? He didn't know you were still listening to him because you weren't looking. You were looking out the window, so he thought you were thinking about something else".

SCIP Phase 2: PRAG 2

PRAG 2.2 Understanding speaker roles

Activity 1: Asking wh– questions

Purpose and target

To help the child to construct wh– questions to gain information and to understand and answer wh– questions.

Materials

Scenes with people in a variety of locations doing a range of things, e.g., a book that folds out to become a house or Make-a-Scene sets.

Create a set of wh– question words, e.g., who, what, and where on arrow-shaped card and write the rest of the question on a separate card.

Procedure

Set up the house scene or the Make-a-Scene sets to have different objects and people in different places that match your questions.

Explain that the task is to ask and answer questions about the scene.

Model setting up a question by selecting the question word and the end of the question on separate cards and putting them together to make a question the child will be able to answer, e.g., select 'WHO' and 'is in the living room?' to make a question.

Read this aloud and answer it, e.g., "Mummy is in the living room".

Repeat with all other question words to make questions that make sense, and the child can answer.

Use questions that require some inference if useful.

Role-reversal

Ask the child to make the questions for you to answer, support as needed, and observe the child's ability to come up with questions with/without the written cue cards.

Meta-challenge

Repeat again when the child is confident, but this time select a question word and ending that do not match e.g., "*where* is *in* the living room?".

Support the child to identify and correct this choice.

If the child attempted to answer, highlight the question to him and the need to listen to the beginning and end of the question.

Repeat with a selection of questions and scenes until the child can confidently create and answer wh– questions.

Role-reversal meta-challenge

Ask the child to deliberately make incorrect question formations for you to correct.

Talk about the questions and observe the child's insight into how he uses questions or not in class or in conversation.

SCIP Phase 2: PRAG 2

PRAG 2.2 Understanding speaker roles

Activity 2: Asking yes/no questions

Purpose and target

To enhance the child's ability to construct yes/no questions to gain information and be able to understand and answer yes/no questions.

Materials

Create two matching sets of aliens of different colours, sizes, shapes, and with different numbers of arms, legs, eyes, etc., and with different alien accessories such as spaceships, guns, lasers, space helmets.

Words written on cards to help the formation of yes/no question words, e.g., does, is, has, on arrow shaped card and the rest of the question on separate cards as separate nouns and adjectives, e.g., eyes, ears, green, purple, black, big, small.

An envelope or pouch to hide the aliens in.

Procedure

The object of this game is to ask yes/no questions to determine which card the other player has selected. Yes/no questions need to be constructed to eliminate aliens in the game until only one is left. The written words act as support for question formation as needed.

Each person has a complete set of aliens at the start of the game.

Explain that this game is learning how to ask yes/no questions to find things out.

Ask the child to choose one alien from his set and hide it in an envelope while you look away. Put all the others out of sight.

Lay out all your aliens face up on the desk with the question words.

Model asking yes/no questions by selecting an auxiliary to start and then adding adjectives and nouns to make a question, e.g., "Is your alien green?", "Does your alien have a gun?".

Support the child to answer as necessary.

Model how to eliminate the aliens that match the child's answer to each question.

Repeat and model many question forms until you find the selected alien.

Role-reversal

Repeat but this time, you hide an alien, and the child makes the questions for you to answer.

Repeat taking turns to model and allow the child to construct yes/no questions until he is confidently formulating questions to work out the hidden alien.

Try to avoid asking questions that will eliminate as many options as possible in one go unless the child proposes this.

SCIP Phase 2: PRAG 2

PRAG 2.2 Understanding speaker roles

Activity 3: Understanding useful questions

Purpose and target

To enhance the child's ability to ask useful questions in conversation.

Materials

Puppet and selection of miniature people.
Examples of questions to use from the Activity 3 Resource.
Pictures of social scenes related to the questions if necessary.
Toy telephone if needed.

Procedure

Explain that you are going to help the puppet learn how to ask useful questions with his
  friends.
Select one scenario from the Activity 3 Resource and draw a picture to represent it if
  necessary.
Explain what the puppet wants and explain that sometimes the puppet asks a silly question,
  "Let's listen and see if it asks a useful question".
Work through each question and explain why this question will or won't help the puppet get
  what it wants.
Give each of the questions a name, e.g., 'not on topic', 'getting there', 'spot on', 'mixed up
  words', 'ridiculous', etc.
Repeat with additional scenes gradually asking the child to make more decisions and use the
  names you have given for the questions when explaining his answers.

Role-reversal

Ask the child to practise creating useful questions for a few of the scenes. Reinforce that
  these questions are 'spot on'.

Meta-challenge

Ask the child to come up with silly questions that won't help the puppet get what it wants.
  Discuss whether these are 'not on topic', 'getting there', 'mixed up words', 'ridiculous', etc.

Personalisation

Using information from the child's ISCP, include events that are pertinent to the child, including any questions he might habitually use.

SCIP Phase 2: PRAG 2

Resource

PRAG 2.2 Understanding speaker roles

Activity 3 Resource: Understanding useful questions

Monkey wants to know if his friend will come with him to these events. He gets on the telephone, and he says ...

Monkey goes to lunch

Not on topic	Do you want to come for a haircut?
Getting there	Are you hungry?
Ridiculous	How many fingers have you got?
Spot on	Do you want to come out to lunch with me?
Mixed up words	You lunch are?

Monkey goes to the park

Not on topic	Do you want to go to the dentist?
Getting there	Do you like playing on the swings?
Ridiculous	What is nine times seven?
Spot on	Do you want to come to the park with me?
Mixed up words	Park you come?

Monkey plays out at playtime

Not on topic	What are you doing at the weekend?
Getting there	Are you a fast runner?
Ridiculous	How many animals can you name?
Spot on	Do you want to play a chasing game with me?
Mixed up words	Chasing you play want?

Monkey is in the library looking for books on space

Not on topic	Have you read all of these books?
Getting there	I like Outer Space, do you?
Ridiculous	How old are you?
Spot on	Do you have any books about Outer Space?
Mixed up words	Outer Space you have book?

It's Monkey's birthday

Not on topic	Do you want to go to the shops?
Getting there	Do you like birthday cake?
Ridiculous	How long can you balance on one leg for?
Spot on	Do you want to come to my birthday party?
Mixed up words	Birthday do you want?

Use miniature people for the next set of questions

John wants to join in with show-and-tell

It's time for show-and-tell. John wants to tell his teacher that he got a kitten yesterday.

He puts up his hand and says ...

Not on topic	Can I go to the toilet?
Getting there	Do you like cats?
Ridiculous	Can you say the alphabet backwards?
Spot on	Can I tell you what I did yesterday?
Mixed up words	Did yesterday I?

Ben wants to ask for more milk

Ben wants more milk for his supper.

He says to his Mum ...

Not on topic	What are we having for breakfast?
Getting there	How much milk do you have?
Ridiculous	Can you do star jumps?
Spot on	Can I have more milk please?
Mixed up words	Milk please more?

Jacob gets picked up from school

Jacob wants to know if his Mum is picking him up from school today.

He says to his Mum ...

Not on topic	Do you think you can run faster than me?
Getting there	Are you working today?
Ridiculous	Can I drive a lorry?
Spot on	Are you picking me up from school today?
Mixed up words	Today school picking?

Anne's lunch

Anne wants to know what sandwiches her Mum has made.

She says to her Mum ...

Not on topic	Can I have corn flakes for breakfast tomorrow?
Getting there	Do you like making cheese sandwiches?
Ridiculous	How many days until Christmas?
Spot on	What sandwiches have you made for us?
Mixed up words	Sandwiches made you?

SCIP Phase 2: PRAG 2

PRAG 2.2 Understanding speaker roles

Activity 4: Understanding multiple questions

Purpose and target

To help the child to develop metapragmatic awareness of the impact of multiple questions on the interaction and to understand that the function of asking questions is to obtain useful information.

Materials

Two puppets.

List of questions.

Pictures of social scenes related to the questions if necessary.

Child's Book of Feelings from work in SUSI 2.

Procedure

Explain that you are going to help one of the puppets learn how to ask questions.

Select one question from the list and set out the matching picture.

Explain what the puppet wants to know and explain that sometimes the puppet keeps asking the same question over and over again and doesn't listen to the answer.

You provide both voices for the demonstration.

Start with the first puppet asking one question, "What's your name?", and the second puppet answers. Make the first puppet ask the same question again. The second puppet gives a matched answer, e.g., "I told you. It's Jamie".

Repeat the question three more times and each time Jamie answers he gets more annoyed and shows this until the last time when he ignores the question.

Discuss Jamie's feelings and why he ignored the first puppet's question.

Repeat but this time with the child answering questions from the first puppet.

Discuss what it is like to answer the same question over and over again.

Relate to SUSI work on feelings and draw this out as a story in the child's Book of Feelings and explain that it has a sad/frustrated ending.

Discuss how to make it better (just ask once and listen to the answer) and draw this out as a happy ending.

Draw the sequence of questions and answers in two columns with an arrow between each question and answer. Draw the arrow returning to the same answer from repeated questions and give this a name, e.g., 'stuck in a loop', a 'sticky question', etc.

Meta-challenge

Ask the child to come up with questions and repeat asking the same question so that the puppet feels annoyed or ignores him.

Personalisation

Using information from the child's ISCP, include events that are pertinent to the child, including any questions he might habitually use.

SCIP Phase 2: PRAG 2

PRAG 2.3 Giving information

Activity 1: Giving clear messages

Purpose and target

To enhance the child's ability to give clear messages and develop metapragmatic awareness of how to simplify information for the listener.

Materials

Simple craft activity with instructions and images at different stages of construction OR a Playmobil scene with photos of the set in at least five stages of construction and one of the final Playmobil scene as you want to make it.

Some instructions and photos that are complicated or impossible.

Procedure

Explain that you are going to take it in turns to make the object or construct the scene by giving each other instructions.

Start the child off by showing the first step picture and giving the instruction that matches, e.g., "Put the rabbit in the garden under the tree".

Show the picture and discuss how it matches what you asked the child to do.

Repeat with one more instruction and start to take turns when the child knows what to do and can tell you what to do from the remaining photos.

Each time discuss that you know what to do because the instruction was clear.

Repeat with the child giving all the instructions for you to follow.

Use natural opportunities to give feedback to the child on how to make the instruction clearer.

Meta-challenge

As the game progresses, introduce the complicated or impossible instructions and observe whether the child attempts to complete them, asks for clarification, or does nothing. Ask, "Do you know what to do?"; "Did you understand that instruction?".

Support him to explain that the instruction is too complicated, and he needs to ask for clarification and simplification. Demonstrate breaking the information down into steps and give one piece of information at a time. Discuss how this helps because it is clearer and simpler.

Discuss how important it is to give clear information and to check whether the other person has understood what has been said. Make a note of how to break instructions down and what to ask when confused.

SCIP Phase 2: PRAG 2

PRAG 2.3 Giving information

Activity 2: Responding to requests for further explanation

Purpose and target

To help the child learn to respond to requests for explanations and to develop
metapragmatic awareness of how to simplify information for the listener.

Materials

Craft activity or Playmobil scenes as in Activity 1.
Long and complex written instructions within the child's reading ability.

Procedure

NB This is a complex activity and will need time to practise.

Following from Activity 1, explain that you are going to take it in turns to give instructions
to make up the object or scene but without photos to guide the construction. Prime the
child by explaining that not having photos will make it harder so we need to help each
other by giving clear instructions and asking if we are not sure.

Start the child off by giving an instruction that they can follow, e.g., "Give the man a spade
and put him under the tree".

Repeat with a second instruction using words the child will not know, e.g., "Put the radishes
in the last row of the allotment".

Support him to ask for explanation about why the instruction was too hard – "It had a new
word that you don't know, or that was too long".

Demonstrate how to simplify the instruction to make it easy to understand: Break it into two
parts, explain the meaning of the words, use a word the child already knows, etc.

Repeat with a few more questions and model what the speaker must do when the listener
does not understand. Support the child to tell you what he does understand and what he
doesn't understand.

Each time reflect that changing the instruction helped him to understand.

Use any naturally occurring misunderstandings to reinforce this skill.

Role-reversal

Repeat, with the aim of the child giving all the instructions for you to follow. If he can read, prepare some written instructions in advance.

Ask him to make the instructions hard for you so that you can ask him for help.

Show confusion and ask for explanation and simplification.

Support the child to simplify the instructions, e.g., "Just tell me one thing, tell me what pieces I need before telling me what to do with them", etc.

Model breaking the information down into steps and allow the child to practise giving one piece of information at a time.

SCIP Phase 2: PRAG 2

PRAG 2.4 Developing metapragmatic awareness

Activity 1: Metapragmatic awareness of conversation conventions

Purpose and target

To help the child to explicitly identify conventions in conversation, and to understand how to react when conventions go wrong.

Materials

Conversation 'rules' written or drawn on separate cards from work in PRAG 2, e.g., look at the speaker, take turns to talk, ask 'good' questions, listen to the answer, not looking at the speaker, repetitive 'sticky' questions, unclear messages, talking at the same time, asking mismatched questions.

Conversation topic cards from Schubi Combimage or other suitable pictures to signal topic.

Speech bubble sticky notes.

Miniature people.

Procedure

Explain the task: "Today we're going to think about the ways in which conversations can be tricky and people sometimes need help to make the conversations go well. We are going to think of all the ways we can help them get it right".

Lay out all the 'rule' cards and explain that to have a good conversation we need to remember all the rules. Each rule card should correspond to a conversational convention that you want to include. This process may be staggered to start with easy conventions and then introduce harder ones later. Select one topic and get the conversation going without convention breaking. Early in the conversation, break one of the conventions and observe the child's response, e.g., deliberately avoid looking at the child and make this very obvious. Stop the conversation and show the 'rule break' card. Talk about the way that this rule break interrupted the conversation.

Draw a picture of one person looking away and the other looking confused and thinking, "Is he talking to me or someone else?". Draw a thought bubble to indicate what the other person is thinking when the mix-up occurs. Write some ways in which this affects the interaction and the other person's response. Discuss with the child what went wrong, why, what to do about the rule break, and what he can do next time in the conversation.

Repeat with more examples of different rule breaks to teach vocabulary to describe and discuss solutions. Illustrate the conversations and the rule breaks on speech bubbles and draw a picture to indicate the thoughts and feelings of the other person. For example, when modelling an interruption, put one speech bubble on top of the other to show the impact; no-one is listening, both are talking, etc. Discuss emotions and use facial expressions related to the impact of conversation conventions and breakage. Focus on solutions and keep a record for the child in his workbook. Observe which skills the child needs additional support with and add to the Phase 2 Planner.

Role-reversal meta-challenge

Ask the child to deliberately make a conversation rule break and discuss the impact on you, confusion, irritation, etc. If the child is reluctant to make a rule break, discuss why and develop his insight into conversational conventions in preparation for Activity 2.

SCIP Phase 2: PRAG 2

PRAG 2.4 Developing metapragmatic awareness

Activity 2: Metapragmatic awareness of conversation conventions (personalised)

Purpose and target

To help the child to explicitly identify the conventions he uses in conversation, and to understand how to modify those conventions in his own conversation.

Materials

Conversation rules from Activity 1.
Conversation topic cards from Schubi Combimage or other suitable pictures.
Picture of the child's interests and favourite topics from his ISCP.
Speech bubble sticky notes.

This activity needs to be sensitively managed, preferably when a strong alliance has been established and the child is robust enough to cope with direct feedback.

Procedure

Explain the task: "Last time we talked about the ways in which people sometimes get mixed up when they are talking, and we came up with some good ideas to help them get it right. Let's do some more about that today".

Lay out the conversation rule cards. Select one topic and get the conversation going. Allow the conversation to flow until it reaches a natural conclusion. Stop the interaction and discuss it in terms of rules used and how they helped the conversation.

If the child makes a rule break, pause and show the facial expression practised in Activity 1 and wait to see if he can modify the talk from this non-verbal cue. If not, use the vocabulary practised in Activity 1 and explain what has happened, e.g., "I am feeling confused now because you are walking away and I don't know if you are still listening/talking to me. Walking away makes me think that you are finished talking to me". Write the conversation down as before, but this time add the impact on the other person.

Ask the child to start again and repeat the same conversation. Say, "Let's try that again and this time let's try to remember our rule for where we stand when talking to show that we are listening and interested".

Repeat with other topics to establish the child's awareness of his strengths and give feedback on skills used and how this helps the conversation be enjoyable for both.

Meta-challenge

Repeat and this time, make conversation rule breaks for the child to notice and comment on.
If he does not notice and gives no response, stop and ask the child to reflect with you.
Explain what you did and how it affected the conversation.

PRAG 3 Intervention content table

SCIP Phase 2	PRAG 3 Intervention content table

PRAG 3 Understanding information requirements

PRAG 3 Information

PRAG 3.1 Understanding impact of missing information

1 Understanding the concepts of a lot, enough, and not enough

2 Missing information in a story

3 Minimal answers in conversation

4 Missing information and requests for clarification

5 Using yes/no questions to check information

PRAG 3.2 Understanding impact of too much information

1 Understanding the concept of giving a lot of information

2 Giving the game away

3 Long answers

4 A lot of questions

PRAG 3.3 Understanding matching context and talk

1 Understanding the concept of matching context to talk

2 Understanding the impact of mismatched context and talk

3 Matching speech acts to context

4 Known and not-known information

5 Matched and mismatched information in conversation

PRAG 3.4 Understanding information requirements in personal conversation

1 Understanding information requirements (personalised)

SCIP Phase 2: PRAG 3

Information

PRAG 3 Understanding information requirements

The purpose of this Section is to help your child understand the concepts of giving information to the listener in conversation. Work in this Section builds on skills introduced in PRAG 2 and aims to further develop your child's understanding of how providing information impacts the listener's ability to follow the conversation. An understanding of what information is shared and does not need to be stated is covered so that your child begins to understand the metapragmatic concept of what information is known to other people.

He will understand the consequences of 'a lot', 'enough', or 'not enough' information for understanding what someone is talking about. Links between people's feelings and receiving information will be covered. Your child will understand the impact of minimal answers on conversation. Strategies to replace guessing about the meaning of missing information will be taught such as using yes/no questions to ask for clarification and check information.

The focus is on developing awareness of these skills and their impact on the interaction. Specific words and phrases will be taught to help your child talk about and think about his/her own conversation skills.

Drawings and other visual representations for information rules will be used to help your child understand and discuss them. Your child will be taught specific vocabulary for information in conversation.

Recent actual conversations with your child will be used to help them reflect on what they do well and what they need to practise.

How you can help

Teaching in this Section will be tailored to meet your child's needs. Please provide information from your child's recent actual experiences of conversation. Please provide information on the words that your child will be familiar with for talking about information requirements in conversation, e.g., "you already told me that" or "you need to tell me more, I don't know where you were or who was there", etc.

SCIP Phase 2: PRAG 3

PRAG 3.1 Understanding impact of missing information

Activity 1: Understanding the concepts of a lot, enough, and not enough

Purpose and target

To help the child to understand the concepts of a lot, enough, and not enough as an introduction to understanding the concept of information in talking.

Materials

Pictures of occupations including a footballer, decorator, and teacher.
Cards with the phrases 'a lot', 'enough', and 'not enough'.

Procedure

Introduce one of the occupations and talk about what the person does, e.g., a footballer. Draw one football and discuss what he can do – he can kick it into the goal, dribble, etc.

Add lots of footballs to the picture. Explain that he now has a lot of footballs and discuss what the footballer will do now. Explain that because he has many footballs, he doesn't know which one to kick.

Show the 'a lot'/'many' cards and discuss what happened.

Explain the link between having a lot of footballs and how the person feels.

Repeat with no football and discuss consequences associated with this, e.g., he can't join in, doesn't know what to do.

Show the 'not enough' card and discuss what happened.

Talk about the link between not enough of something and how the person feels.

Repeat with other occupations, e.g., the decorator has many pots of paint, or not enough; the teacher has a lot of whiteboards covered in writing.

Ask the child to join in as soon as he can to explain what happens and use the phrases 'a lot' and 'not enough'.

SCIP Phase 2: PRAG 3

PRAG 3.1 Understanding impact of missing information

Activity 2: Missing information in a story

Purpose and target

The child will understand the consequences of missing information on comprehension of the whole story.

Materials

Pictures to represent the main ideas and events from fairy tales or simple stories that the child will know well.

Script for each story that leaves out key events or people.

Procedure

Arrange one set of pictures from one of the stories but leave out one main idea or person.

Go through the pictures one at a time and tell the story leaving out the 'missing' information.

Stop at the end and ask the child if he followed the story. Ask if there was anything missing.

Discuss with the child the piece of information that was missing if he does not spontaneously comment on it.

Talk about the idea of missing information and the confusion it causes.

Help the child to draw the missing character or event and add this to the story so that it is complete.

Re-read the story and discuss that the added information makes the story better and the listener doesn't feel confused anymore.

Repeat with another well-known story and engage the child in spotting the missing information and in repairing it as before.

Role-reversal

Give the child a set of pictures with some missing information to arrange a story and ask him to tell the story.

Observe his reaction to the missing information, does he add it in, leave it out, or comment that it should be included.

If he leaves it out, demonstrate feeling confused. Ask a question that reflects the confusion, e.g., "How did Goldilocks get into bed? You didn't tell me she went upstairs to bed".

Explain how the missing information is misleading, e.g., "I thought she fell asleep at the breakfast table. I got that wrong. I was confused. I imagined her asleep with her head on the table next to the porridge", etc.

Discuss that sometimes people will forget to tell all the information and we need to listen carefully and ask if we are confused. Reinforce the words, not enough information and confusion, and make a note in the child's workbook.

SCIP Phase 2: PRAG 3

PRAG 3.1 Understanding impact of missing information

Activity 3: Minimal answers in conversation

Purpose and target

To help the child understand the impact of minimal answers on conversation.

Materials

Puppet.
Pens and blank cards to write rules for information.

Procedure

Explain that the puppet is learning how to answer questions by giving just enough information and not too little. Explain that the puppet has been to a film or outing and you would like to find out about it.

Start a conversation with the puppet who gives you minimal answers so that the conversation doesn't flow, and you don't get the information you need.

For example: Q: "What happens in the film?". A: "Lots of things". Q: "Is it a funny film?". A: "Yes".

Talk about what happens when the puppet doesn't give you the information you need, i.e., you don't know if you would like that film or not.

Write down some rules on the blank cards for the puppet to follow, e.g., tell the start of the film, tell who was in it, where it was set, what the people did, etc. and repeat with the same question so the puppet can follow the rule and give enough information.

Discuss how these rules helped and repeat with another set of questions about another event.

Role-reversal

Involve the child in asking some questions to the puppet and give minimal answers for the child to correct the puppet. Support the child to explain what the puppet should do to give a better answer.

Write down the words the child uses to explain what the puppet should do and use these as a new rule.

Role-reversal meta-challenge

Ask the child to act for the puppet and give minimal answers to questions from you. If the child is reluctant to do this, discuss why and develop his insight into providing information if needed in preparation for PRAG 3.4.

SCIP Phase 2: PRAG 3

PRAG 3.1 Understanding impact of missing information

Activity 4: Missing information and requests for clarification

Purpose and target

To help the child understand how requests for clarification can be used to ask for missing information.

Materials

Playmobil sets or similar play scenarios.

Examples of requests for information written on separate cards, e.g., I don't know what to do; you didn't tell me XX, etc.

Examples of complete instructions on where to put characters and objects and some with missing information, e.g., "put the boy wearing the _____ on the swing".

Procedure

Explain the task as setting up a Playmobil scene to play with and that you will give instructions that the child can follow and some that will have missing information.

Read aloud the examples of requests for information and place them on the table and explain that these will help when he needs to ask for more information.

Start with a few simple and clear instructions to get the Playmobil set started.

Give an instruction that is too vague to understand completely.

If the child guesses, allow him to complete his action and then pause to allow the child to notice this and ask for clarification.

If the child doesn't respond to this non-verbal prompt, say, "Did you understand? I don't think so. You didn't understand because I left something out, didn't I? So, if you are not sure, don't guess, you need to ask for more information".

Select a matching request for clarification from the set.

Repeat the instruction and prompt the child to make the request for clarification.

Reply and give the information needed and praise the child for asking and allow the child to complete the action accurately.

Repeat with at least six more instructions, half of which should have missing information or until the child has stopped guessing and is spontaneously asking for information to complete the task.

Write some examples of requests for clarification in the child's workbook.

SCIP Phase 2: PRAG 3

PRAG 3.1 Understanding impact of missing information

Activity 5: Using yes/no questions to check information

Purpose and target

To help the child use yes/no questions to ask for clarification and check information.

Materials

Alien characters, e.g., Manic Martians from the Manic Martians game.

Magnetic Way, Fuzzy Felt, or Make a Scene reusable sticker sets.

A list of instructions to make a picture.

A set of nonsense words for the alien to use.

Procedure

Explain that a Martian has landed on earth, and it wants to play with us today when we make a picture using our sticky pictures or fuzzy felt.

Start by asking the first Martian, "What would you like to make a picture of?" Martian replies in Martian (you use nonsense words) and no-one can understand him.

Explain to the child that we can ask questions to help us work out what he wants. Explain we can offer a choice. Ask the Martian, "Do you want to make a boat on the river or a house with a garden?".

The Martian gives a long answer in Martian. No-one knows what he wants. Explain that the choice question didn't help, it was too long.

Explain that we need to ask a simple question and get the Martian to say just 'yes' or 'no' by asking a yes/no question, e.g., "Would you like to make a farm?".

Martian turns his back on the speaker. Discuss that this might mean he's not interested.

Ask another question and make the Martian jump up and down with excitement.

Explain that this means that he means 'yes' and start building the picture.

Repeat by asking the Martian, "What do we need next?" so that the Martian replies in Martian.

Repeat with a choice question and discuss that we still don't know because we asked the wrong question.

Help the child formulate a yes/no question to find out and discuss how the simple yes/no question was helpful.

Repeat and ask questions in this way until you have built the picture.

Talk about why we needed to check what he wanted and what helped and what didn't help. Explain that, when we don't have all the information we need, we can ask questions to check and that yes/no questions can help us to understand.

SCIP Phase 2: PRAG 3

PRAG 3.2 Undestanding impact of too much information

Activity 1: Understanding the concept of giving a lot of information

Purpose and target

To help the child understand the consequences of giving a lot of information during conversational interactions.

Materials

Simple play street map.

Cars/trucks in different colours.

Red traffic light card saying 'STOP! Information overload!'.

Green traffic light card saying 'OK, I understand!'.

Procedure

Introduce the activity as a game about following instructions and listening carefully.

Start the game by giving two simple instructions, e.g., make the red car park outside the bank.

Next give a really long instruction with overly precise details and ask the child to do the action.

When the child cannot succeed or doesn't attempt the instruction, talk about the difference between the two instructions. "So, some instructions seem easy, and some seem very long".

Explain that when there is a lot of information, we feel confused because there is too much to listen to.

Give some more examples and ask the child to tell you which instructions contain too much information by using the traffic light sign to show you when too much information is being given.

Include instructions that give extraneous information, such as the blue car *with four doors and four wheels and a windscreen*.

Talk about the consequences of being given a lot of information – you forget, you get confused, you can't keep up with it all, you don't need to know all that information.

Role-reversal

Repeat and this time ask the child to give you instructions. Ask him to give good instructions and some that are too long.

Demonstrate confusion and make mistakes in following the long instructions.

Discuss how the long instructions caused you to feel confused and not sure what to do. Reinforce the phrase 'too much information'.

If the child is reluctant, discuss why and develop his insight into his own ability to provide information if needed in preparation for PRAG 3.4.

Create some rules for giving information and write some examples of requests for clarification in the child's workbook.

SCIP Phase 2: PRAG 3

PRAG 3.2 Understanding impact of too much information

Activity 2: Giving the game away

Purpose and target

To help the child understand the consequences of giving a lot of information during a game-based interaction.

Materials

Guess Who game or similar barrier game activity.

Puppet who doesn't understand the game and keeps giving the answers.

Red traffic light card saying 'STOP! You're giving the game away!'.

Green traffic light card saying, 'OK, I understand!'.

Procedure

Introduce the activity by saying that you are going to play a guessing game with the puppet. Explain to the puppet that the child doesn't know/can't see the picture and the point of the game is not to tell the answer.

Play the Guess Who game with the practitioner acting for the puppet.

When the puppet gives the right answer, show the green card and say, "Well done, that was just right".

When you are sure that the child understands the game, make the puppet give too much information when the child asks a question, e.g., "Yes, it is a man, and he is wearing glasses".

Observe the child's reaction and talk about what went wrong, e.g., "You told me it was Charlie. I wanted to work it out. Now the game is spoiled".

Show the red card to the puppet and say, "You gave away the game by giving too much information".

Repeat this several times using the traffic lights to praise or stop the puppet.

Role-reversal

Reverse roles to allow the child to give answers to the puppet's questions and instruct him to answer only Yes or No.

Observe if the child unwittingly gives a lot of information and use the traffic light cards as before.

Provide feedback on all the child's answers.

Role-reversal meta-challenge

Ask the child to deliberately give the game away by adding extra information to the answer and discuss the impact on the game as before.

If the child is reluctant to join in, discuss why and develop his insight into information giving if needed in preparation for PRAG 3.4.

SCIP Phase 2: PRAG 3

PRAG 3.2 Understanding impact of a lot of information

Activity 3: Long answers

Purpose and target

To introduce the child to the metapragmatic concepts of giving long answers and saying just enough.

Materials

Questions written on cards.

Microphone for television interview.

Red traffic light card saying 'STOP! That's a lot of information!'.

Green traffic light card saying 'OK'.

Puppet.

Child's Book of Feelings.

Procedure

Introduce the activity as taking turns to interview each other for a TV show: "I am a television interviewer and I want to find out about the puppet". Tell the child, "Your job is to listen to the answers and stop him if his answers are too long. You can hold up the traffic light cards".

Start the interview by asking questions and the puppet gives good answers.

Then the puppet starts to give very long verbose answers. Encourage the child to use the traffic lights to stop the interviewee going on too long.

When the child is successful at identifying when to stop the answer, ask, "Why did you have to use the red traffic light? When did you use the green traffic light? How did that feel when you had to listen to all that talking?".

Discuss the feelings associated with listening to too much information: Bored, confused, didn't understand, stopped listening, switched off. Refer to the Book of Feelings as needed.

Agree rules about how much people say and write these down in the child's workbook.

Involve the child now and help him to ask the puppet some questions.

Repeat the long and 'just enough' answers and support the child to spot when the puppet is talking a lot, if needed.

Role-reversal

Reverse roles and set the child up as the interviewee and the puppet asks the questions. Observe if the child unwittingly gives a lot of information and use the traffic light cards as before. Provide feedback on all the child's answers and discuss their answers with him, e.g., "Why did I have to use the red traffic light? When did I use the green traffic light? How did it feel when I told you there was a lot of talking?". Write down feelings related to too much information in the workbook and cross reference to the Book of Feelings.

Role-reversal meta-challenge

Ask the child to deliberately give long answers and discuss with him what happens when he does this. If the child is reluctant to do this, discuss why and develop his insight into information giving if needed in preparation for PRAG 3.4.

SCIP Phase 2: PRAG 3

PRAG 3.2 Understanding impact of too much information

Activity 4: A lot of questions

Purpose and target

To assist the child to understand the effects of asking too many questions during an interaction.

Materials

Pictures of social situations that might lead to a policeman asking lots of questions, e.g., bike having been stolen; mum has lost her keys.

Fox puppet or similar figure.

Policeman figure.

Red traffic light card saying, 'STOP! That's a lot of questions!'.

Green traffic light saying, 'OK, good question!'.

Procedure

Describe what is happening in one of the pictures and introduce the policeman. Explain that he asks the characters in the story questions about what they saw, where they were, did they see anyone else, etc. Name these questions as a 'good question'.

Demonstrate this as the child listens and use the green traffic light card to show that the policeman is asking just enough questions.

Introduce the curious fox puppet and act for the puppet to ask a lot of questions using the same story and characters. Ask the child to raise the red traffic light card when multiple questions are being asked.

Talk about what happened, e.g., "Who asked a lot of questions?".

Discuss the impact of a lot of questions on how someone feels and write these down or draw facial expressions.

Reverse roles and allow the child to ask the questions.

Observe the child's questions and provide feedback on whether he is being like the policeman or the fox – asking just enough or a lot of questions.

Draw up some summary rules about asking questions and put these in the child's workbook.

Role-reversal meta-challenge

Ask the child to deliberately ask a lot of questions and discuss with him what happens when he does this. If the child is reluctant to do this, discuss why and develop his insight into information giving if needed in preparation for PRAG 3.4.

SCIP Phase 2: PRAG 3

PRAG 3.3 Understanding matching concept and talk

Activity 1: Understanding the concept of matching content to talk

Purpose and target

To help the child begin to understand the metapragmatic concept of matching what is said to the physical and language context.

Materials

Topic cards: These show an event or people dressed for, or engaged in, different roles (use scenes from sequence sets).

Create a set of idea cards with speech acts written on them, which are a mixture of matched and mismatched information for that topic or person role.

Make two cards marked 'YES, it goes with this' and 'NO, it doesn't go with this'.

Procedure

Say, "Today we're going to think about things that belong together and things that don't belong together. We are going to sort these ideas to see if they go with the pictures or not. Let's have a look at this picture first". Present first event picture and explain it.

Set out the two cards marked Yes and No. Say, "Now I'm going to make two lists – ideas that go with the picture and ideas that don't go with the pictures".

Start with a familiar picture and obvious examples of matched and mismatched ideas, e.g., "This man is a postman, he will talk about parcels and letters. He might say, 'here is your parcel'".

Make sure that you explain clearly whether this idea goes with or doesn't go with the picture.

Continue to work through the cards and pictures, sorting the ideas. Give clear reasons why the ideas are matched or not and use a repetitive phrase to establish this, e.g., "This man is a painter. He will talk about painting and things he needs for painting. He won't talk about cooking things. This idea is about cooking. It doesn't belong".

After demonstrating a few, pause after reading the idea to allow the child to join in and decide whether the idea goes with the picture or not.

Once the child has got the idea of the game, repeat all from the beginning, telling the child to sort them out as you read the ideas.

Ask the child to give reasons and scaffold these using the same familiar phrases. If the child is confident on the first run through, use the words matched and mismatched and ask the child to use these as well.

Draw up some summary rules about matching content to talk and put these in the child's workbook.

Role-reversal meta-challenge

Ask the child to deliberately suggest mismatched ideas for each picture. If the child is reluctant to do this, discuss why and develop his insight into using mismatched information if needed in preparation for PRAG 3.4.

Personalisation

Introduce to the game mismatched comments that you have heard the child make and observe his response.

SCIP Phase 2: PRAG 3

PRAG 3.3 Understanding matching context and talk

Activity 2: Understanding the impact of mismatched context and talk

Purpose and target

To help the child understand the impact of matched and mismatched information on comprehension (simple).

Materials

Two puppets.

Red traffic light sign saying 'STOP!'.

Cards marked 'YES, it goes with this' and 'NO, it doesn't go with this' from Activity 1.

Stories matched to child's age and interests.

Create a list of matched and mismatched comments on cards for each story.

Procedure

Say, "Today we're going to see what happens when people talk. Sometimes they say things that belong in the story (matched) and sometimes they say things that don't belong in the story (mismatched). I've got two puppets – one is a good talker and can tell a good story that goes together and makes sense. But the other one sometimes says things that don't go with the story and gets the ideas mixed up".

Demonstrate one puppet telling a short story and saying only things that are matched to the narrative.

Next demonstrate with the same story using the other puppet to say some things that are matched and some things that are mismatched. Stop after the mismatched comment and ask the child to hold up the STOP sign. Suggest that the puppet could stop talking about the mismatched idea and get back to the story. Explain that the mismatched information is confusing.

Ask the child to listen again and this time he is to hold up the STOP sign when he hears the mismatched comments. Support as needed.

Explain the impact of the mismatched comments: "I was confused; I thought a spaceship had landed in the park. Why did he talk about lorries in the story about the beanstalk?". Explain some possible reasons; for example, he was thinking about his favourite things, he wasn't paying attention. Talk about how to fix it, "just keep talking about the story". "This story isn't about lorries", etc.

At the end of that story, write down what each puppet said and use red and green pens to tick and cross matched and mismatched comments if this is helpful.

Repeat for four more stories, observing the child's response to the mismatched comments and ask the child to explain the reasons and suggest how to fix it. Observe if the child shows any insight into his own use of mismatched comments.

Role-reversal and role-reversal meta-challenge

Ask the child to tell the story using both the matching and non-matching puppets. If the child is reluctant, discuss why and develop his insight into his use of information if needed in preparation for PRAG 3.4.

SCIP Phase 2: PRAG 3

PRAG 3.3 Understanding matching context and talk

Activity 3: Matching speech acts to context

Purpose and target

To help the child understand the impact of matching and mismatching information in speech acts.

Materials

Pictures of social situations showing at least two people who could be talking, e.g., Schubi Tell Me About It sequence sets or ColorCards: Skills for Daily Living: Social Behaviour Daily Living.

Speech bubble sticky notes; red and green pens.

Ideas for matched and mismatched exchanges between two characters in the scenes.

Procedure

Following from Activity 2, say, "Today we're going to see what happens when people talk to each other. Sometimes they say things that belong in the conversation (matched) and sometimes they say things that don't belong in the conversation (mismatched), just like in the stories".

Start with a familiar picture and obvious examples of matched and mismatched ideas.

"This boy is at the ice cream shop. He says to the man, 'Can I have an ice cream please?'. The man says, 'Yes. What flavour do you want?'". Say, "These belong together".

Write these down on the sticky notes and stick them on the picture or write them on a sheet of paper or in the child's workbook. Add another comment that is mismatched from the boy, e.g., "Do you like spaceships?" Write these down and talk about how the man feels [confused]. Does he know what flavour the boy wants? What will happen? Will the boy get the flavour he likes?

Explain the impact of the mismatched comments.

Repeat with a second scenario and continue to work through the pictures changing the position of the mismatched idea in the conversation.

Role-play some scenes. Explain that you are now going to pretend to be the people and have a chat. Get the conversation going and keep matching. Stop to talk about the comments being matched.

Meta-challenge

Start again and add a mismatched comment. Observe the child's response. If he carries on talking and doesn't respond to the comment, stop the role-play and write down the conversation, including the mismatched comment and discuss.

Role-reversal meta-challenge

Ask the child to deliberately suggest mismatched ideas for each conversation. If the child is reluctant, discuss why and develop his insight into information giving if needed in preparation for PRAG 3.4.

Personalisation

Introduce the child's common mismatched comments to the conversation and observe his response.

SCIP Phase 2: PRAG 3

PRAG 3.3 Understanding matching content and talk

Activity 4: Known and not-known information

Purpose and target

The child will understand the metapragmatic concept of what information is known to other people.

Materials

Two figures or puppets.

Up to ten pictures of different objects and a large, coloured envelope to hide them in.

I know/I don't know cards from work completed in Phase 1 CM.

Two sets of three clues about the pictured objects (providing a hint of what the object might be) written on separate cards for each object, and blank cards.

Procedure

Explain that we are learning about what people know and what they don't know. Explain that often different people know different things.

Set out the two figures and explain that one object picture has been hidden in the envelope.

Say, "No-one knows what the picture is yet", and give each character an 'I don't know' card

In order to work it out, the characters need some information

Give one character the first clue and the other character a blank card. One clue does not give it away.

Explain that one clue is not enough and repeat, giving the same character another clue and give the same second clue to the second character.

Repeat until one character has all three clues and the other, only one. Show that the character with all the clues can work it out. Give this character an 'I know' card.

Talk about the character with only one clue – she still doesn't know. She is confused and can't play. She needs more information.

Support the child to give the clue cards one at a time to the second character until she too can work it out. Swap her card to 'I know' when she can work it out.

Explain that as they were playing, the characters knew different things and use phrases like, 'not everyone knows that', 'he doesn't have that information'.

Repeat for all ten picture cards or until the child has shown an understanding of different people having different information and how this impacts on their ability to work things out and play the game.

Meta-challenge

Use very obviously mismatched clues and explain that these don't help to work it out, e.g., clue one: 'This is a vehicle'; clue two: 'This person is happy'. Support the child to notice that these clues don't go together, and they should match. Use words and phrases from activities in this Section and discuss how mismatched information makes the game more confusing for everyone.

SCIP Phase 2: PRAG 3

PRAG 3.3 Understanding matching context and talk

Activity 5: Matched and mismatched information in conversation

Purpose and target

To help the child to understand how to distinguish between matched and mismatched information in conversation.

Materials

Questions requiring some verbal reasoning, e.g., "Why does a dog make a good pet?" from *Verbal Reasoning Activities* by J G DeGaetano (or similar).

Write a set of matched and mismatched reasons on cards for each question.

Procedure

Explain that we are learning about matching reasons and not-matching reasons and we're going to talk about different ideas and try to give reasons to go with each question.

Start with "Why does a dog make a good pet?".

Present the reasons one at a time and discuss as you sort them into matching reasons and not-matching reasons.

Say, "So if we said, 'Because he is fun to play with', that would be a matching reason. But if I say, 'It has legs', that would be a not-matching reason".

Explain that this is because it doesn't tell you anything about how the dog behaves as a pet.

Continue through the rest of the reasons allowing the child to suggest reasons when he is clear about the game.

Repeat with the other questions, e.g., "Would a tiger make a good pet?".

Finish each picture with a revision of the matching and not-matching reasons.

Repeat at least five times until the child can join in recognising and reflecting on the reasons.

Role-reversal meta-challenge

Ask the child to deliberately suggest not-matching reasons for each set of questions. If the child is reluctant, discuss why and develop his insight into using information if needed in preparation for PRAG 3.4.

SCIP Phase 2: PRAG 3

PRAG 3.4 Understanding information requirements in personal conversation

Activity 1: Understanding information requirements (personalised)

Purpose and target

To help the child develop the metapragmatic ability to monitor his own use of matched and mismatched information in conversation and begin to self-correct.

Materials

Cards marked 'YES, it goes with this', and 'NO, it doesn't go with this'.

Cards marked 'a lot', 'not enough', and 'just right'.

Stories matched to child's age and interests.

Information from the child's ISCP on common mismatching comments in conversation.

Procedure

Say, "Remember our puppets sometimes said things that belonged in the story (matched) and sometimes they said things that didn't belong in the story (mismatched). Today, we're going to tell each other a short story from these pictures. Sometimes it will be a story that goes together and makes sense, but sometimes it will have things that are out of place, and which don't go with the story, and sometimes it won't have all the ideas we need to make a good story. We will listen carefully and say, 'Stop' when we hear something that doesn't belong or when we are confused. I'll go first". Start the story and say only things that are matched to the narrative. Ask the child if he understood the story. Discuss why it was easy to follow.

Meta-challenge

Start a new story and add mismatched ideas. Pause to allow the child to decide whether the idea goes with the story or not. Prompt him to notice the mismatched comment and discuss why it doesn't match, using phrases practised in this Section, e.g., 'It doesn't belong', etc.

Repeat with another story leaving out important information and discuss as before.

Role-reversal and role-reversal meta-challenge

Ask the child to tell a story and instruct him to include only ideas that are matched to the story.

Pause to comment on the ideas and praise the child for talking about only the matched ideas.

Pause after any mismatched comment and show signs of confusion. Discuss and come up with solutions.

Ask the child to introduce deliberately mismatched comments into his story. Support by pointing to things on the page or in the room that he could use as a mismatched idea. Make this fun. Repeat, this time supporting the child to leave out important information.

Discuss the impact of not/talking about things that are important in a story.

Personalisation

Repeat and tell a new story using any mismatched comments the child commonly uses. Observe to see if the child shows any insight or recognition of these phrases and note what he says and if he tries to correct you.

Discuss the impact and find a few phrases that the child can learn to expect to hear from others in response to mismatched comments and record these phrases in the child's workbook.

PRAG 4 Intervention content table

SCIP Phase 2	PRAG 4 Intervention content table

PRAG 4 Understanding and managing topic in conversation

PRAG 4 Information

PRAG 4.1 Identifying topics

1 Identifying topic in narratives

2 Identifying favourite topics

3 Understanding how to move between topics

PRAG 4.2 Understanding topic change conventions

1 Signalling a topic change

2 Identifying and repairing topic changes

PRAG 4.3 Consolidating topic skills

1 Understanding mismatched topics

2 Understanding mismatched topics (personalised)

SCIP Phase 2: PRAG 4

Information

PRAG 4 Understanding and managing topic in conversation

The purpose of this Section is to help your child understand the rules of topic management in conversation and to be able to introduce and change topics in conversation. The Section starts by teaching how to listen closely to the words (in a story) in order to work out what topic is being discussed. Your child will be taught some phrases to use to change topic explicitly, e.g., 'and then'/'well that was the first thing that happened'/'I want to tell you another thing too', or to recognise that a pause in the conversation might indicate that a new topic is coming up. Drawings and other visual representations for topic change rules will be used to help your child understand and discuss them.

The Section then goes on to teach that everyone has a favourite topic that is related to his/her own interests. Activities teach that it is important to be able to talk about a range of different topics. An understanding of the consequences of talking too much about one topic in conversation will be taught. Links between people's feelings and talking at length on one topic will be covered. The aim is to help your child to understand the impact of choosing topics in conversation.

This Section teaches your child to identify topic changes as a means of developing awareness of his/her own use of topic change markers. Role-play and puppets are used to show topic conventions. Topic change markers in conversation rely on being aware of subtle signs that the speaker is interested or bored, has lots to say, or not very much to say on a particular topic. When he has understood the basic rules of topic change, your child will learn how to look out for topic changes made by puppets or the speech and language therapy practitioner in role-play.

Work in this Section builds towards your child being able to reflect on his/her own topic management skills. The focus is on developing awareness of these skills and the impact their use has on the interaction. Specific words and phrases will be taught to help your child talk about and think about his/her own conversation skills and topic management behaviour.

Recent actual conversations with your child will be used to help him reflect on what is done well and what he needs to practise.

How you can help

Teaching in this Section will be tailored to meet your child's needs. Please provide information on the words that your child will be familiar with for talking about topic in conversation and provide ideas for topics that your child likes to talk about.

SCIP Phase 2: PRAG 4

PRAG 4.1 Identifying topics

Activity 1: Identifying topic in narratives

Purpose and target

To help the child be able to identify topics in stories, to understand that the 'topic' is 'what is being talked about', and to use the word topic in metapragmatic discussions.

Materials

Short narratives with a clear topic theme.
Topic cards showing a picture or word for the topic of each story, e.g., Schubi Combimage.

Procedure

Explain the game and say, "We're going to listen to a short story and then we're going to say what the story is about. That is called the topic". Stories and conversations have a topic. We need to know what the topic is in stories and when we are talking to people.

Set out two or three topic cards and start to read the first story.

Ask the child to select the card that matches the topic of this story.

Say, "That's right, the topic of this story is a broken-down car. That is the topic. Let's see if you can show me the topic for the next story".

Read the second story. Repeat the identification process and support the child to use the word 'topic' when telling you what the story is about, e.g., "Can you tell me, 'The topic is …'".

Talk about the words in the story that help identify the topic, e.g., "You heard me say Zookeeper. The topic is a day at the Zoo". Write the topic and the key words in the child's workbook using a word-web layout.

Repeat at least five times and keep reinforcing the idea of being able to identify the topic by listening to the words. Reinforce the word 'topic' and link it to stories and conversations.

Try a few stories without providing a topic card as a cue. Support the child to identify the topic if needed and show the topic card after it has been identified correctly.

Discuss the words in the story that help work out the topic.

Write a definition of a topic as 'something we talk about' in the child's workbook. Add some of the topics the child could work out and draw or write the clue words from the story that helped identify the topic.

SCIP Phase 2: PRAG 4

PRAG 4.1 Identifying topics

Activity 2: Identifying favourite topics

Purpose and target

To help the child learn about the metapragmatic concept of a favourite (or preferred) topic as something people like to talk about a lot. The child will identify favourite topics for himself and others.

Materials

Occupations cards to include a footballer and an IT engineer or person at a PC.
Topic cards matched to each person's occupation and matching short narratives.
A drawing of yourself and the child and blank cards to draw personal favourite topics.
Ideas for the child's favourite topics from the ISCP.

Procedure

Explain that some people have things that they like to talk about a lot. This is their favourite topic. This game is to work out who likes to talk about each of the topics.

Say, "We're going to listen to a short story and see if we can work out who would like to talk about this topic".

Set out some occupation cards and read the first story. Help the child to match the topic card to the person. Repeat with all occupations and support the child to use the words 'favourite topic' when telling you which person matches to the story. Talk about why they like talking about this topic – they're good at it, it makes them feel relaxed, they feel happy when they talk about it.

Now set out the favourite topic cards and the occupations cards face down on the desk and play a matching pairs game. As each pair is matched, repeat, "That's right, that is his favourite topic". As a mismatched pair is turned, say, "No, he wouldn't like to talk about that at all; that's not his favourite topic and he might be bored".

Personalisation

Build on the idea that everyone has a favourite topic by drawing a picture of yourself and a few favourite topics for you. Support the child to draw a picture of himself and a few things he likes to talk about. Add these to the existing set of topics and people and play another pairs game. Repeat the phrases, "That's right, that is his favourite topic" and

"No, he wouldn't like to talk about that at all, that's not his favourite topic and he might be bored", to reiterate ideas of interest and boredom with other people's favourite topics. Write a definition of a favourite topic as 'something we talk about a lot'. List the child's favourite topics in his workbook.

SCIP Phase 2: PRAG 4

PRAG 4.1 Identifying topics

Activity 3: Understanding how to move between topics

Purpose and target

To help the child learn the metapragmatic concept of talking about different topics. The child will learn how people can talk about different topics.

Materials

Occupations cards to include a footballer and an IT engineer or person at a PC.

Topic cards matched to each person's occupation.

Drawings of yourself, the child, and favourite topics created in Activity 2.

Procedure

Following from Activity 2, introduce the activity as follows: "Last time we talked about favourite topics, and we found out that different people have different favourite topics. Your favourite topic is, e.g., Mario. Now we're going to mix up the topics between the people. It's important to do that because even if you have a favourite topic, you can learn how to talk about other things too".

Set out the people and topic cards including yours and the child's.

Select two people and one of their favourite topics and say, "We're going to see if this person can talk about this topic. It's not his favourite, but he can try. Let's think about what he could say".

Take both roles and get a conversation going between the people. Model questions and answers and comments for both speakers.

Say, "He did well; he talked about someone else's favourite topic. He asked a question and listened". Repeat with one more mixed pair and model simple question formats that can be applied to all topics, e.g., "Tell me about painting. What do you like to paint?" Repeat and ask the child to take on one of the talking roles.

Now engage the child talking about his favourite topic. Explain that it is not your favourite, but you can ask questions and listen. Talk about how it went. How did he feel when you asked a question and listened to the answer? Explain, "That is called showing an interest in your friend".

Ask the child to join in talking about a topic that is not his favourite using either yours or the other characters' topics. Talk about how it went. "Did you ask and listen?", "Was it OK?".

Continue the role-play until the child can ask a question and listen to the answer for a few different topics. Explain, "So we've shown that even if you have a favourite topic, it's easy to talk about other topics too".

Write a list of the topics the child could talk about in the child's workbook along with some standard questions that can be asked of any topic.

Meta-challenge

In a role-play with the child on a topic they can talk about, but not their favourite topic, don't ask any questions and show a bored face. If the child doesn't notice and comment, pause and ask if the conversation is going well, if you are asking and listening, etc. Encourage the child to give advice to you on how to ask to show you are interested and listen to be friendly, and how this makes the other person feel.

SCIP Phase 2: PRAG 4

PRAG 4.2 Understanding topic change conventions

Activity 1: Signalling a topic change

Purpose and target

To help the child to be aware of and use accepted topic change conventions.

Materials

One puppet who will 'learn' topic change behaviours.

Topic change phrases and behaviours written on cards: 'And then'/'Well that was the first thing that happened'/'I want to tell you another thing too'/Pause/Take a breath.

Procedure

Explain that we are learning how to change from one topic to another in a conversation. Explain as follows: "I'm going to talk about two things that I did yesterday. These are the two things that happened. I'm going to write them down and use them as topics".

Write these events down or draw two pictures to represent them.

Start talking about the first topic and then suddenly switch to the second topic for two sentences with no warning.

Say to the child and the puppet, "Did you see how I swapped from that topic to this topic really quickly?". Explain that it is confusing to have two topics at the same time. Say, "We have to do something in between the topics. We have to show that we have finished with one topic and are starting another. Here's one way we can change from one topic to another".

Insert a topic change behaviour card in between the two topic cards.

Say, "Now I'm going to do that again, but this time, I'm going to do this change in the middle. Listen carefully and see what I do". Repeat the activity but clearly demonstrate the topic change behaviour to the child and the puppet.

Repeat with all topic change behaviours. Ask the child to listen carefully and tell you which one you used.

If the child needs to observe more times, ask the puppet to show him how to do it.

Role-reversal

Repeat and ask the child to have a go at talking about two topics and showing the change. Write two things that the child did recently on two cards and lay them on the table. Ask the child to start talking about one and then select a topic change card to say before he starts the next topic.

Support by offering to point to the cards in turn so that the child starts and moves and stops on your cue.

Repeat with at least two more topics and use all topic change behaviours.

SCIP Phase 2: PRAG 4

PRAG 4.2 Understanding topic change conventions

Activity 2: Identifying and repairing topic changes

Purpose and target

To help the child to learn how to identify when topic change rules are broken; and to develop awareness of his own use of topic change markers.

Materials

Same puppet who learned topic change behaviours in Activity 1.

A new puppet who doesn't know the topic change rules.

Topic change cards from Activity 1.

Procedure

Following from Activity 1, explain that we have a new puppet who needs to learn how to change from one topic to another in a conversation. Revise the topic rules and introduce the puppet.

Ask the child to be the teacher and help the puppet to learn the new rules.

Ask the child to set out two topics for the puppet to talk about.

Act for the puppet and start talking about one thing that he did yesterday. Make sure the child is listening as you make a sudden topic change with no topic change marker.

Observe the child's reaction. Does he notice, comment, not notice? Pause to discuss and ask the child what happened? Encourage the child to explain that the puppet did not show that he was changing topic/use the rule/made me feel confused, etc.

Ask the child to give advice to the puppet and support the child, if needed, to put a topic change card in between the new puppet's topic cards.

Act for the puppet to repeat and this time, use the topic change card.

Discuss with the child that his advice helped the puppet to follow the rules and make the conversation better. Ask the child to explain again to the puppet that it is confusing to have two topics at the same time and not show that you have changed your topic.

If needed, add a visual reward, e.g., the child gets a star on a chart for having a good idea about how to make the conversation better.

Repeat with a few different topics and show the puppet sometimes following the topic change rule and sometimes making a sudden switch of topic. After each topic shift, pause to allow the child to give feedback to the puppet on what they did well and what they need to do to make it better.

Support the child as needed to say, e.g., "Don't jump from one topic to the other. Tell me that you have a new topic. You should say, 'and then'", etc.

Role-reversal meta-challenge

Introduce a third puppet and ask the child to act for this puppet who doesn't know the rules. Ask him to talk about the topics and not include a topic change comment and explain that the other puppets will help him.

SCIP Phase 2: PRAG 4

PRAG 4.3 Consolidating topic skills

Activity 1: Understanding mismatched topics

Purpose and target

To help the child learn to identify mismatched topics in talk and the effect they have on interaction.

Materials

Counters or tokens.

Schubi Combimage cards for topics.

Puppet who has not yet been used in learning topic change rules.

Procedure

In this activity, the practitioner and the child talk about the story together and stay on the topic of the story. Explain, "We are learning how to stay on the topic that has been chosen in a conversation".

Give each person and puppet a pile of tokens. Explain as follows, "Let's talk about this story. This story is about swimming. That's the topic we have chosen today".

Say, "We're going to talk about the story in these pictures, but if we talk about something else, we will lose a token. Let's see who has the most tokens at the end. They will have done a good job of staying on topic. When we stay on the chosen topic, we have a good conversation".

Start your discussion about the story, taking turns to talk about it, as in Activity 2. After a little while, act for the puppet and interrupt with a different topic that has nothing to do with the story. Stop to listen and then say, "Oh dear, that isn't what the story is about, you are talking about a different topic. Sorry, that means you lose a token". Ask the puppet to think about the topic and to join in with the conversation by saying something about swimming.

Make the puppet interrupt a few times quickly in a row, each time with a different topic. Repeat the phrases, 'that's a different topic' and 'think about this topic' regularly so the child can hear them and use them to advise the puppet.

The puppet interrupts again and this time look to the child to see if he has noticed and encourage him to give advice to the puppet. Stop to discuss what happened and why it is important to have only one topic of conversation at a time.

Repeat with a new story and make the puppet interrupt with the same words and the same topic three or four times in each story. Repeat the phrases as above, and add, 'you really want to talk about XX' and 'sorry, we are not talking about XX at the moment'.

Continue until the puppet has lost all tokens. Count up the tokens and see who has the most and who has none left. Explain why the puppet lost his tokens. Say, "Because he didn't talk about the story; he was talking about other things; he was talking about different topics".

Discuss how it feels to be interrupted by different topics, e.g., bored, fed up, annoyed.

Role-reversal meta-challenge

Ask the child to act for the puppet and to interrupt with different topics. If the child is reluctant, discuss why and develop his insight in preparation for Activity 2. In discussion, revise all metapragmatic vocabulary taught in this Section and review the importance of listening to the other person and allowing them time to talk, talking about the topic, and talking about favourite topics as well as topics we don't like so much.

SCIP Phase 2: PRAG 4

PRAG 4.3 Consolidating topic skills

Activity 2: Understanding mismatched topics (personalised)

Purpose and target

To help the child establish metapragmatic awareness of his own use of topics in interaction and to be able to change these with personalised guidance.

Materials

Cards with your and the child's favourite topics created in PRAG 4.1 Activity 2.

Schubi Combimage cards for other topics.

Puppet and a few favourite topic cards for the puppet.

Blank cards to develop personalised guidance for topic changes.

A list of the child's individual topic behaviours from observation and from report on the child's ISCP.

Procedure

For round one, set out three topic cards in this order: Schubi topic card on top, then the practitioner's favourite topic, and, on the bottom, the child's favourite topic.

Explain, "We are going to talk about all of these topics in order. Let's start with this one and then we will move to the next topic and then the next".

Say, "I'm going to talk about this topic. You listen for a while and then I'm going to change to the next topic and then I'll pick up the next card and talk about that topic. You see if I can get it right". At the end say, "It was hard to switch from my favourite topic but it's better to talk about lots of topics, not just my favourite".

Repeat using the puppet and place his favourite topic in the middle. When the puppet gets to his favourite topic, he produces the child's typical behaviour, e.g., he doesn't move on, gives too much information.

Discuss with the child what is happening. Agree what the impact of the behaviour is and what the puppet needs to do. Write this on the card, e.g., move on, don't talk so much about lorries, can you try a new topic? etc.

Allow the puppet to have another go and repeat making a different topic behaviour, e.g., listing facts, moving to the new topic but then switching back to the favourite topic, talking only briefly on the first topic to get to the favourite quickly, etc. Discuss and record possible changes and guidance as before.

When you are confident that the child can identify his own behaviour and has heard the solutions, let him have a go. Put his favourite topic in the middle of the two other topics. Discuss how things went and ask the child to evaluate too. Give feedback and let the child practise a few times until you are satisfied that he can identify his own topic behaviours and can use his personal guidelines developed in this activity.

Role-reversal meta-challenge

Ask the child to act for the puppet and deliberately break some of the topic rules you have developed. If the child is reluctant, discuss to determine and develop his insight into his use of this topic and what would help to make a change in his reliance on this topic. Write up in the child's workbook.

PRAG 5 Intervention content table

SCIP Phase 2	PRAG 5 Intervention content table

PRAG 5 Understanding and improving discourse style

PRAG 5 Information

PRAG 5.1 Understanding different styles in interaction

1 Understanding features of conversation style: Polite and formal

2 Understanding features of conversation style: Friendly and polite

3 Understanding styles for known and not-known people

4 Practising conversation styles

5 Mismatches in conversation styles

PRAG 5.2 Understanding and using conventions of interaction style

1 Focus on greetings

2 Focus on invitations

3 Focus on farewells

4 Understanding indirect speech acts plus Resource

5 Using indirect speech acts

PRAG 5.3 Consolidating interaction style

1 Identifying mismatches in style plus Resource

2 Identifying mismatches in style (personalised)

SCIP Phase 2: PRAG 5

Information

PRAG 5 Understanding and improving discourse style

The purpose of this Section is to help your child understand how to adapt interaction style to suit the situation and people he is talking to. The Section starts by teaching vocabulary for the features of conversational style such as politeness, proximity (how close you stand), and formal versus informal styles of interaction. Your child will learn about why it is important to interact differently with known and not-known people. Drawings and other visual representations for interaction style rules will be used to help your child understand and discuss them.

The Section then goes on to teach that sometimes we don't always match our talk to a situation or people – we can all do this. Links between other people's feelings and these mismatches will be covered, e.g., confused and irritated. We aim to help your child begin to understand the impact of style mismatches in conversation and will introduce him to a set of ways to monitor and change style.

There is a particular focus on understanding the conventions for greetings, farewells, and invitations. The Section contrasts polite and impolite styles of interaction and teaches how to understand and make indirect requests as a further polite style of interaction. Understanding indirect requests uses drawings of what people are thinking, contrasted with what they are saying and shows how what they say is interpreted by the listener.

Throughout this Section your child will be asked to identify mismatches as a means of developing awareness of his/her own skills and needs. Through role-play and using puppets to show mismatches, your child will understand the impact of these in conversation. Work in this Section builds towards your child being able to reflect on his own skills. Specific words and phrases will be taught to help your child talk about and think about his own conversation skills.

Recent actual conversations with your child will be used to help them reflect on what is done well and what he needs to practise.

How you can help

Teaching in this Section will be tailored to meet your child's needs. Please provide information from your child's recent actual experiences on how he typically performs in conversation. Please provide possible situations and words that your child will be familiar with for talking about how to adapt interaction style to suit the situation he is in.

SCIP Phase 2: PRAG 5

PRAG 5.1 Understanding different styles in interaction

Activity 1: Understanding features of conversation style: Polite and formal

Purpose and target

To help the child understand and identify features of conversational style such as politeness, formality, and proximity: adult interlocutors.

Materials

Labels for conversational styles: Starting the conversation/how you talk to people you know/ how you talk to people you don't know/how close do you stand?/being polite/what you talk about.

Characters to represent a woman, a man, a shopkeeper, or similar occupation.

Procedure

Explain the task: "Today we're going to talk about the ways in which people talk to each other. Sometimes when we talk to a grown-up, we talk in a different way to the way we would talk to a friend. We're going to pretend to be different people and have a conversation. Let's pretend to be grown-ups, first of all. We're going to listen and then we will talk about the different ways people talk to each other".

Present the mother and shopkeeper characters and put the first label, "Starting the conversation" on the table between them. Role-play a conversation referring to each conversation label as you act out the exchange of buying food for the barbeque. Show the characters following the rules.

Comment on the fact that Mum and the butcher don't know each other well and so they will talk in a certain way, which is different from the way you would talk to your friends. Explain that this is called polite and formal. At the end, review each aspect of the conversation as modelled.

Meta-challenge

Repeat the role-play with a man coming into the shop who breaks the rules. Refer to each style label as the role-play progresses using the rule breaks below and discuss, e.g.,

❖ what should the man say when he goes into the shop? "Hiya mate" or "Hello Mr Forest"?

❖ what would the shopkeeper say? "Good morning, how can I help you?" or "What do you want?"

❖ would the man stand next to the shopkeeper, or would he stay on this side of the counter?

❖ would the man say, "Can I have 6 sausages, please?" or "Give me the sausages now!"

❖ would the man say, "Can I have 6 sausages please?" or "Can I have some sunglasses and a hat?"

As you role-play each step, explain the ways you styled the conversation in terms of language, posture, formality, words used, proximity and topics, using words and phrases the child can understand and adapt the style labels to suit. Discuss solutions as you progress.

SCIP Phase 2: PRAG 5

PRAG 5.1 Understanding different styles in interaction

Activity 2: Understanding features of conversation style: Friendly and polite

Purpose and target

To help the child understand and identify features of conversational style such as politeness, formality, and proximity: child interlocutors.

Materials

Labels for conversational styles: Starting the conversation/how you talk to people you know/ how you talk to people you don't know/how close do you stand?/being polite/what you talk about.

Characters to represent two children.

Procedure

Following from Activity 1, explain that we are going to look at how children speak to each other when they are friends. Remind the child to listen to the children talking and think about how they are speaking and what they are doing.

Present the two child characters and put the first label, 'Starting the conversation' on the table. Explain that the children are friends, and they are meeting in the playground after the holidays.

Role-play a conversation referring to each conversation label as you act out the exchange of catching up with each other after the holidays.

Comment on the fact that the children know each other well and so they will talk in a certain way, which is different from the way you would talk to adults or people you don't know. Explain that this is called friendly and polite. Review each aspect of the conversation as modelled.

Meta-challenge

Repeat the role play with one child now breaking the rules. Refer to each style label as the role-play progresses using the rule breaks below and discuss, e.g.,

❖ what should the friend say first? "How are you, Sam?" or "Hi Sam, how was your holiday?"

❖ what should the friend say? "Thank you for asking", or "Hi Jack, I had a great time"

❖ would you say, "Where did you go on holiday?" or "I'm really bored with you!"

❖ what should the friends talk about? "My dog is a terrier", or "We went to Disney World."

❖ should they stand next to each other or leave a big gap between them?

As you role-play each step, explain the ways you styled the conversation in terms of language, posture, formality, words used, proximity and topics, and using words and phrases the child can understand and adapt the style labels to suit. Discuss how friends would talk to each other and contrast with Activity 1 using matching vocabulary, e.g., friendly/casual/informal. Discuss looking at and passing each other things to look at so you need to be close enough to see what you are sharing, etc. Discuss why this distance is the right distance for friends. Explain that we tend to stand further away from someone we don't know so well.

SCIP Phase 2: PRAG 5

PRAG 5.1 Understanding different styles in interaction

Activity 3: Understanding styles for known and not-known people

Purpose and target

To help the child become familiar with the features of conversational style for interacting differently with known and not-known people.

Materials

Labels for conversational styles from Activities 1 and 2.

Pictures or name cards for the child's immediate family, friends, and classmates.

Pictures of famous people, TV actors, and authority figures.

Pictures of unknown adults and children.

Four labels: I know these people really well/I know these people quite well/I know something about these people, but I don't know them in real life/I don't know these people.

Procedure

Explain the task: "Today we're going to talk about the ways in which people talk to each other when they know them and when they don't know them".

Start by sorting the people into the four categories and support the child to sort as needed.

Clarify any confusion as to familiarity and relationship by explaining the relevant factors when making the decision:

❖ does he know the person's name?

❖ does he play with the person?

❖ has he visited this person at home?

❖ is this person on TV?

Now set up a role-play, taking the role of one character from each box in turn and the child acts as himself. Using the style labels, model a style-matched conversation with the child for at least one character from each box, e.g., the child's brother, a friend at school, a teacher, and a stranger. Explain the importance of changing how we speak depending on how well we know someone and let the child practise a few times for each group of people.

Meta-challenge

Repeat the role-play with the child acting as himself and act out being overly friendly as a stranger to the child and overly formal when playing with a known person. Discuss the mismatch and how it made the child feel. Explain that sometimes mismatches happen and discuss the impact of these briefly.

Role-reversal meta-challenge

Ask the child to deliberately make some style mismatches for you to identify. If the child is reluctant, discuss to determine and develop his insight into his use of style changes in preparation for activities in PRAG 5.3.

SCIP Phase 2: PRAG 5

PRAG 5.1 Understanding different styles in interaction

Activity 4: Practising conversation styles

Purpose and target

To assist the child to develop awareness of how people speak to each other differently depending on who they are and to suit the social context they are in.

Materials

Labels created for conversational styles from previous activities in PRAG 5.

Pictures of different social situations, e.g., dining room, classroom, playground, assembly, café, swimming pool, Scout clubroom, etc.

Laminated pictures of adults and children to represent parents, friends, teachers, strangers, etc.

A blank page with two columns of at least four blank speech bubbles to represent four turns for each person.

Procedure

Explain the task: "Today we're going to practise talking in different ways to different people". Name the styles as they are written on the cards and use matching vocabulary.

Select two children and the playground and model an interaction for the people and the setting, e.g., "Come on, play football with us", "OK I'm coming", "hurry up", "pass the ball", "I can score", etc.

Stop and write each turn on to the speech bubble sheet (using one column for each speaker).

Show the relevant style cards and ask the child to check if you have recorded it correctly.

Repeat this scene and ask the child to join in and make contributions for one of the characters. This can be very close to what was just modelled if necessary.

Now, select a different context and using the same children explain that they will speak to each other differently because they are in a different situation, e.g., in class, politely asking for equipment, "Can I have the ruler when you have finished?" and not, "give that here", etc.

Repeat a few times using pairings of equal status and model polite, friendly, formal, casual, etc.

Repeat using a pairing of unequal status and discuss in detail as before and how changing the situations influences what the characters say to each other.

Use scenarios of strangers meeting in different contexts, at a party, asking for directions in the street, etc. and take time to discuss and reflect with the child why the style changes are important.

Meta-challenge

When the child is confidently joining in and evaluating the interactions accurately, model mismatches of style for the child to detect and correct. Discuss styles and impact of styles on people's feelings and move to Activity 5.

SCIP Phase 2: PRAG 5

PRAG 5.1 Understanding different styles in interaction

Activity 5: Mismatches in conversation styles

Purpose and target

To help the child develop awareness of how people use different styles of verbal interaction to match the relationship and the context.

Materials

All materials as for Activity 4 with completed conversations written out.
Speech bubble sticky notes.

Procedure

Following from Activity 4, explain the task: "Let's look at the conversations we made last time and think about what happens when people sometimes get their way of talking mixed up".

Take a completed conversation and add one sticky note to illustrate a style mismatch for one interlocutor only, e.g., being too polite with a friend.

Now act this conversation out with the child. Make it fun while exaggerating your response to the mismatch and explaining it while in character, e.g., "Hey, Danny, why are you speaking to me like I am the Headteacher? That's way too formal for us. You can speak to me like a friend. You can just say 'Hi'".

Discuss the mismatch and the impact on the other person's feelings.

Repeat a few more mismatches between pairings of equal status before using a pairing of unequal status. Alter the scenes and the pairings to provide the child with the opportunity to identify a range of mismatches and suggest ways to modify these.

As the child understands the purpose, provide fewer clues as to the mismatch being added and observe his response when you make a mistake. Does he notice it, attempt to repair it, tell you the style rule you have broken?

Personalisation

Include style mismatches that the child himself has used in a meta-challenge and observe how well he can identify and offer advice for changes. Probe to see what insight the child has developed in this area, e.g., ask, "Has that ever happened to you?".

Role-reversal meta-challenge

Ask the child to make a mismatch of style for a character in the role-play for you to identify.

SCIP Phase 2: PRAG 5

PRAG 5.2 Understanding and using conventions of interaction style

Activity 1: Focus on greetings

Purpose and target

To help the child understand conventions associated with greetings linked to relationships and context.

Materials

List of situations familiar to the child where greetings are required (e.g., playground, birthday party, Scouts, Brownies, etc.). Use pictures if necessary.

Child and adult characters: Playmobil figures or laminated pictures of people.

Names of familiar adults and friends.

Examples of his own ways of greetings from the child's ISCP.

Procedure

Explain the task: "Today we're going to talk about the ways in which people say hello to each other. Sometimes we say hello in different ways depending on whom we are talking to. Let's pretend to be different people and say hello to each other".

Use two characters to model a greeting between friends in a playground. Add a teacher, 'Miss Chalk', to the scenario and ask the child to suggest how the children should greet the teacher. Model some situation-matched phrases and discuss the difference between greeting friends and greeting people in authority.

Repeat using figures to represent different people (e.g., familiar adults, authority figures, friends, new child at school) in different situations (e.g., classroom, playground, birthday party, cafe).

Repeat for a few different people and situations. Discuss and explain different greetings and their importance using words and phrases the child can understand, as in previous work in PRAG 5.1.

Meta-challenge

When the child is confidently joining in and evaluating the greetings, accurately model mismatched greetings for the child to detect and correct. Discuss the impact of these mismatches on people's feelings.

Personalisation

Include any mismatches noted in the child's ISCP in the meta-challenge and observe how well he can identify and offer alternatives. Probe to see what insight the child has developed in this area, e.g., ask, "Has that ever happened to you?".

Role-reversal meta-challenge

Ask the child to use the figures to role-play making greetings mismatches and discuss the impact of using a mismatched greeting, how people might feel, what they might say or do.

SCIP Phase 2: PRAG 5

PRAG 5.2 Understanding and using conventions of interaction style

Activity 2: Focus on invitations

Purpose and target

To help the child understand pragmatic conventions associated with invitations linked to relationships and context.

Materials

List of situations familiar to the child where invitations are required (e.g., playground, birthday party, school play, sporting events). Use pictures if necessary.

Child and adult characters: Playmobil figures or laminated pictures of people.

Names of familiar adults and friends.

Blank cards for invitation rules (event, reason, invitation).

Procedure

Explain the task: "Today we're going to talk about invitations. An invitation is when we ask someone to do something with us or to join in with an activity or game. Let's pretend to be different people and invite each other to do something".

Explain the 'rules' for making an invitation – explain the event, explain the reason, and make the invitation. Write these down on the blank cards. Use the characters to model an invitation between friends as follows: Explain the event, why it is important to the child, and add a request to join in. Say, "I am in my school play this year (event). I am playing one of the Seven Dwarves and I tell a joke (reason). Would you like to come to watch me in the school play? (invitation)". Point out that you followed the rules. Repeat for a few different people and situations, including asking someone to play or work together in school. Start role-play for each new situation with the child responding to the invitations you model.

Role-reversal

Ask the child to select a character and an event and role-play with the child creating an invitation based on the rules/steps practised. Use scenarios and people you have practised if needed.

Meta-challenge

Repeat a few more invitations but leave out one of the three rules. Observe the child's response to the omissions and talk about why the invitation didn't work.

Personalisation

Include examples reported from the ISCP and a familiar social context in a role-play. Observe how well he can identify and suggest changes. Probe to see what insight the child has developed in this area, e.g., ask, "Has that ever happened to you?".

Role-reversal meta-challenge

Ask the child to make deliberate mismatches in invitations and explain what he missed out and the impact on the other person.

SCIP Phase 2: PRAG 5

PRAG 5.2 Understanding and using conventions of interaction style

Activity 3: Focus on farewells

Purpose and target

To help the child understand pragmatic conventions associated with farewells linked to relationships and context.

Materials

List of situations familiar to the child where farewells are required (e.g., playground, birthday party, school play, sporting events). Use pictures if necessary.

Child and adult characters: Playmobil figures or laminated pictures of people.

Names of familiar adults and friends.

Examples of farewells from the child's ISCP.

Procedure

Explain the task: "Today we're going to talk about saying goodbye to different people in different ways". Use two characters to model a typical farewell between friends in a playground. Add a teacher, 'Miss Chalk', to the scenario and ask the child to suggest how the children should say goodbye to the teacher. Model some context-matched phrases and discuss the difference between saying "See ya" to a friend and saying "Goodbye Miss" to the teacher. Talk about giving a 'high five' or a hug to a friend, but not to a new/ unknown child or a grown-up.

Repeat using figures to represent different people (e.g., familiar adults, authority figures, music or dance tutors, friends, new child at school) in different situations (playground, birthday party, Brownies, gym lessons, swimming pool) and include conventions for each, e.g., "Thank you for coming to my party", "See you at school on Monday", etc.

Repeat for a few different people and situations.

Meta-challenge

Set up a role-play and make mismatches in farewells including ignoring the other person and mismatched styles. Observe the child's response and ask him to give you advice on how to improve it.

Personalisation

Include examples reported from the ISCP and a familiar social context in a role-play. Observe how well he can identify and suggest changes. Probe to see what insight the child has developed in this area, e.g., ask, "Has that ever happened to you?".

Role-reversal meta-challenge

Ask the child to make deliberate mismatches in farewells and discuss the impact on the other person. Ask him to explain what was missed out and what the solution is. If the child is reluctant, discuss why and develop his insight in preparation for Objective 5.3 Activity 2.

SCIP Phase 2: PRAG 5

PRAG 5.2 Understanding and using conventions of interaction style

Activity 4: Understanding indirect speech acts

Purpose and target

To help the child develop awareness of how people use indirect speech acts as a form of politeness.

Materials

Create the scenes and written texts as described in the Activity 4 Resource.

Cards with polite, rude/impolite and indirect/hidden written on them.

Sticky notes for thinking and speech bubbles.

Procedure

Explain the task: "Today we're going to talk about some of the ways people can be polite when they are talking". Explain that there are two ways to be polite: Say what you are thinking and use polite words like "please". This is called polite. Explain that another way to be polite is to say something indirect or hidden. Indirect means that the other person has hidden some information so that you have to 'work out' what they mean. Say that being indirect gives a clue to what people want or how they feel. Explain that not being polite is called being rude. Show all three cards and explain that the child needs to listen and decide which card matches what the children are saying to each other.

Start with the first scenario in the Resource and explain what each person wants by referring to the words in their thinking bubbles.

Explain that the person can ask in a polite way, i.e., say the words in the thinking bubble plus 'please' to create a polite direct request. Then discuss the rude request and the impact of the rude request on the other person.

Now talk about asking in an indirect way. Say, "When we give the other person clues so they can work out what we are thinking, we are being indirect".

Take the indirect phrase and stick it on the person who is thinking about asking for something.

Use the space below the picture to write or draw what the person wants and how we know (from their eye gaze and words). For example, I know he wants the cake because he is looking at it and smiling and he said, "That cake looks yummy". Say, "He thinks the cake is yummy. If you like the cake, you will probably want to eat it. I think he wants to eat that last slice of cake".

Discuss in full to ensure the child understands the thoughts and intentions associated with the indirect request, the means of being indirect, and what to expect or how to respond when using an indirect request.

Repeat using a few more examples, including one adult scenario.

Gradually, build up each scenario in turn leaving gaps for the child to fill as they understand the task and learn how to be indirect. Ask the child to write onto the speech and thought bubble sticky notes to gain insight into skill level with this.

To provide variety, mix up the polite, rude, and indirect phrases for each scene and ask the child to sort them out.

SCIP Phase 2: PRAG 5

Resource

PRAG 5.2 Understanding and using conventions of interaction style

Activity 4 Resource: Understanding indirect speech acts

Draw these scenarios on a sheet of paper leaving at least half the page blank:

- ❖ two children looking at one last piece of cake on a plate
- ❖ two children, one playing on a bike, the other watching
- ❖ two children working in class, one child talking or messing around
- ❖ two children playing a game and one looking bored and left out
- ❖ three adults in a room, a window in the background, closed, one person looks uncomfortably warm
- ❖ two women having lunch in a café

Scenario 1

Create a thinking bubble to add to one child's head saying, 'I want the last bit of cake'.

Create three options for what to say as polite, rude, and indirect. For example, "Could I have the last piece of cake, please?", "I'm having that bit of cake", and "That cake looks really delicious".

Scenario 2

Create a thinking bubble to one child's head saying, 'I want to play on the bike'. Create three options for what to say: Polite, "Can I have a turn on the bike, please?"; rude, "Give me the bike"; and indirect, "That looks like lots of fun".

Scenario 3

Create a thinking bubble to one child's head saying, 'I want to do my work'. Create three options for what to say: Polite, "Can you be quiet, please?"; rude, "Shut up"; and indirect, "I can't work with all this noise going on".

Scenario 4

Create a thinking bubble to one child's head saying, 'I don't like this game'. Create three options for what to say: Polite, "Can we play something else now, please?"; rude, "I'm bored with this game"; and indirect, "What other games have we got?".

Scenario 5

Create a thinking bubble to one adult's head saying, 'I want to open a window'. Create three options for what to say: Polite, "Can you open a window, please?"; rude, "Open the window", and indirect, "It's warm in here today, isn't it?"

Scenario 6

Create a thinking bubble to one adult's head saying, 'I have forgotten my purse'. Create three options for what to say: Polite, "Can you pay for me today, please? I have forgotten my purse"; rude, "You can pay for my lunch"; and indirect, "Have you got any spare cash on you?".

SCIP Phase 2: PRAG 5

PRAG 5.2 Understanding and using conventions of interaction style

Activity 5: Using indirect speech acts

Purpose and target

To help the child understand and practice using indirect speech acts and to develop the child's awareness of how people use indirect speech acts as a form of politeness.

Materials

Pictures of social situations that can be used to generate indirect requests, e.g., from Schubi Tell Me About It sequence sets (card 11 can be used for asking to go out on a sunny day; card 9 can be used to ask a friend to play quietly while you read; card 21 can be used to ask for a ride home when your car breaks down).

Cards with polite, rude/impolite, and indirect/hidden written on them.

Sticky notes for thinking and speech bubbles.

Ideas from the child's ISCP on any instances of indirect speech use.

Procedure

Explain the task: "Last time we talked about using indirect requests to ask for things in a polite way. Now we are going to practise asking in this way. Let's look at this picture. The girl has dropped her ice-cream and is upset. She could say to her brother, 'Give me your ice-cream', but that would be rude. She could say, 'Can I have another ice-cream please?'; that would be polite. To be indirect she will say something that will make Mum think, 'Jessica needs another ice-cream'. Jessica could say, 'Oh no, I dropped my ice-cream. I really wanted to eat it.' Mum will be able to work out that she wants another".

Write this on the speech and thinking bubbles as you go through the scenario.

Repeat using a few different scenarios and guide the child to create an indirect request by talking through what clues there are in the picture as to what the person wants and what clues he can give the other person so he can work out what they are thinking.

Personalisation

Use reported situations from the child's ISCP in which he has used direct instead of indirect speech acts. Present a comic strip to represent this scenario and provide options of what to say to be polite, direct, or indirect. Draw it out with the options and explain that this sometimes happens to everyone. Observe the child's reaction to this scenario and ask, "Has that ever happened to you?". As the child recognises the scenario, discuss to determine and develop insight and solutions for this scene.

SCIP Phase 2: PRAG 5

PRAG 5.3 Consolidating interaction style

Activity 1: Identifying mismatches and solutions in style

Purpose and target

To help the child develop awareness of the impact of mismatched interaction styles and develop alternative strategies.

Materials

Scenarios from the Activity 1 Resource which includes examples of how to target mismatches between language use and social situations in:

- ❖ overly honest comments
- ❖ sitting too close
- ❖ too noisy and over-excited
- ❖ talking about fantasy not reality and using a cartoon voice
- ❖ not using intonation

Speech bubble sticky notes.
Book of Feelings or emotion ladders from work in SUSI 2.

Procedure

An example is included in the Activity Resource. Select one scenario that is distant from the child's behaviours before working on ones similar to his needs. As you examine similar scenarios, judge whether he is robust enough to develop insight in this area before moving to Activity 2.

Explain the task: "Today we're going to think about the ways in which people sometimes say something but do another thing". Provide an example.

Present one scenario and write a conversation between the characters to illustrate the selected style mismatch. Write a contribution from each character on speech bubbles and include the mismatch. Draw a thought bubble to indicate what the other person is thinking when the mismatch occurs.

Observe the child's response to the mismatch and if necessary, stop to prompt him to notice the mismatch and think about what impact it will have.

Discuss with the child what happened, why, what to do about the mismatch, and what he can do next time. Write some ways in which this affects the interaction and the other person's response. Add vocabulary to describe what went wrong and the solutions.

Repeat with distant to generic scenarios until the child is ready to work on personal insights.

Explain the impact of words and actions for each mismatch, e.g., say, "Someone will think I am rude if I say, 'you've got silly pink hair'". Say, "Someone might hit me if I say, 'you've got a big nose'". Say, "If I sit too close to Tomas, he won't be able to work".

Repeat with another example of the same mismatch or repeat with a different mismatch until the child is confidently able to identify mismatches in the interaction.

Role-play some scenarios with the child on the receiving end of a mismatch and observe his responses. Discuss the impact and how he felt about what you did or said.

Refer to the child's Book of Feelings or emotion ladders to discuss feelings.

SCIP Phase 2: PRAG 5

Resource

PRAG 5.3 Consolidating interaction style

Activity 1 Resource: Identifying mismatches and solutions in style

Scenario 1: Overly honest

This activity is designed to tackle problems around making comments related to speaking openly without tact and personal comments about people and their appearance or behaviour.

Draw these scenarios on a sheet of paper leaving at least half the page blank:

- ❖ a woman with a very large nose
- ❖ a man with a very large stomach
- ❖ a girl with bright pink and orange hair
- ❖ a boy with a tattoo on his arm
- ❖ a boy wearing a very brightly coloured shirt
- ❖ a boy riding a bike that is too small for him

In all pictures, add another adult or child who is looking at them. Leave space above this person's head to add thinking bubbles.

Start talking about the first picture and explain that sometimes people see things that make them feel surprised or interested. They might think about that, and they might even say something. Let's look at what might happen in this picture.

Adult: What might this girl be thinking? (Point to the second girl who is looking at the woman with a big nose.)

Child: She's got a big nose!

(Draw a thought bubble and write in child's comment.)

Adult: That's right, she's thinking about the girl's nose. The girl might say, "Gosh! What a big nose!".

(Write comment on speech bubble sticky note and stick on picture.)

If she does say that, explain that this is called being 'overly honest'. When you say exactly what's in your head, that is called being overly honest.

Adult: Sometimes being overly honest can make people feel upset, hurt, or embarrassed. How would this girl feel if someone says, "What a big nose you've got"?

(Write emotion onto a sticky note and stick it by the girl.)

Adult: You're right. The girl with the big nose would be embarrassed or upset if her friend was overly honest. What might her friend say if she wanted to be friendly?

Child: Would you like to play with me today?

(Write this onto a speech bubble sticky and replace the mismatched comment.)

Adult: How would the girl with the big nose feel then?

Child: Happy that she's got a friend to play with.

(Replace the 'embarrassed' sticky note with one saying 'happy'.)

Repeat this kind of discussion for each of the style mismatches covered in this Resource: being overly honest, proximity, being over-excited, talking about fantasy worlds, lack of intonation.

Scenario 2: Sitting or standing too close

This activity is designed to tackle needs around proximity with peers/adults in school situations.

Draw these scenarios on a sheet of paper leaving at least half the page blank:

❖ reading with a teacher
❖ working in a group
❖ in the hall for Physical Education lesson with lots of other children
❖ music or choir in the music room
❖ playground or open space

In all pictures, add another adult or child who is being leaned on or squashed by the child who is being too close. Leave space above this person's head to add thinking bubbles.

Start talking about the first picture and explain that sometimes people get too close to the people they are working/playing with and that they can feel uncomfortable. Use context-matched words to explain this idea and work through the stories as set out in Scenario 1.

Scenario 3: Too noisy and over-excited

This activity is designed to tackle problems with mismatches of behaviour and context and in topic management.

Draw these scenarios on a sheet of paper leaving at least half the page blank:

❖ being at school on your birthday, too excited to work, constant chatter about party
❖ working in the library on the computer causes over-excitement
❖ end of term treats make working and concentrating on reading very hard
❖ visitor to the school, waiting for them to come to your class

In all pictures add another adult or child who is being interrupted by the child who is being too noisy and excited. Leave space above this person's head to add thinking bubbles.

Start talking about the first picture and explain that sometimes people get too excited when something good is going to happen. Use context-matched words to explain this idea and work through the stories as set out in Scenario 1.

Scenario 4: Mixing up fantasy and reality

This activity is designed to tackle problems of preferred topics that are in the realms of fantasy, or over-use of scripts from TV in conversation.

Draw these scenarios on a sheet of paper leaving at least half the page blank:

❖ in a café having lunch and talking about the food
❖ in a class discussion about rainforests
❖ talking to a friend about holiday plans

In all pictures, add another adult or child who is confused by the child who is saying unexpected things that sound like a TV show. Leave space above this person's head to add thinking bubbles. Start talking about the first picture and explain that the people are talking about the food and what they like best. Talk about what happened when one person talks about TV shows instead of talking about the food. Use specific words to explain this idea and work through the stories as set out in Scenario 1.

Scenario 5: Not using intonation to show interest and excitement

This activity is designed to tackle mismatches of intonation and context.

Draw these scenarios on a sheet of paper leaving at least half the page blank:

- ❖ winning a prize at school
- ❖ a day at the funfair
- ❖ a birthday party

In all pictures, add another adult or child who is confused by the child who is talking about the event but in a flat tone. Leave space above this person's head to add thinking bubbles. Start talking about the first picture and explain that the people are talking about the exciting thing that has happened. Explain that one child is talking in a way that makes the other person think they are not pleased or interested in the event.

Talk about what happened when one person talks in this way instead of talking and sounding excited. Use context- and person-matched words to explain this idea and work through the stories as set out in Scenario 1.

SCIP Phase 2: PRAG 5

PRAG 5.3 Consolidating interaction style

Activity 2: Identifying mismatches and solutions in style (personalised)

Purpose and target

To help the child to develop awareness of the impact of his own use of mismatches in style.

Materials

Using information in the child's ISCP, create scenarios similar to those in the Activity 1 Resource to include the child's style mismatches and situations in which these are observed.

Pen and paper to draw scenes.

Speech bubble sticky notes.

This activity needs to be sensitively managed, preferably when a strong alliance has been established and the child is robust enough to cope with direct feedback.

Procedure

Explain the task: "Last time we talked about the ways in which people sometimes say and do the things that don't match, and we came up with some good ideas to help them spot the mismatches. Let's do some more work on that today".

Present one scenario and say, "I know that sometimes when you are, e.g., over-excited, you might be too noisy and silly in class. Here is a picture of you in class last week".

Explain how you know what happened, "your teacher told me that XX".

As you draw and write the situation as reported, encourage the child to add information as you work.

Identify together what the mismatch between style and situation was and draw these, adding thought and speech bubbles for all people.

Stop after you write out the mismatch and observe the child's response. Pause to allow him to make any contribution he can before drawing a thought bubble to indicate what the other person is thinking when the mismatch occurs and explain the impact and why the person thinks and feels as they do.

Pause regularly to allow the child to contribute and suggest solutions. Use the vocabulary introduced in Activity 1 to describe the mismatches and solutions.

LANGUAGE PROCESSING (LP) CONTENT TABLES AND INTERVENTION ACTIVITIES

Language Processing (LP)			
Sections	*Objectives*		
LP 1 **Vocabulary and word knowledge**	LP 1.1 Understanding semantic relationships between words	LP 1.2 Consolidation and self-cueing	LP 1.3 Vocabulary enrichment
LP 2 **Narrative construction**	LP 2.1 Understanding inferences in picture sequences	LP 2.2 Telling complex and personalised stories	LP 2.3 Constructing novel stories with plot
LP 3 **Non-literal language**	LP 3.1 Understanding homophones	LP 3.2 Understanding literal and non-literal meanings	LP 3.3 Understanding non-literal meanings in context
LP 4 **Discourse comprehension**	LP 4.1 Improving memory and listening	LP 4.2 Understanding verbal inferences	LP 4.3 Understanding stories
LP 5 **Enhanced comprehension monitoring**	LP 5.1 Text level comprehension monitoring	LP 5.2 Task based comprehension monitoring	

DOI: 10.4324/9781032706641-6

LP 1 Intervention content table

LP 1 Vocabulary and word knowledge

LP 1 Information

LP 1.1 Understanding semantic relationships between words

1 Understanding semantic categories

2 Understanding relationships within categories

3 Understanding salient features of objects

4 Understanding functions of objects

5 Understanding definitions

LP 1.2 Consolidation and self-cueing

1 Understanding word knowledge plus Resource

2 Consolidating understanding of word knowledge

3 Supporting self-cueing in conversation

LP 1.3 Vocabulary enrichment

1 Understanding synonyms plus Resource

2 Understanding antonyms plus Resource

3 Dictionary skills plus Resource

SCIP Phase 2: LP 1

Information

LP 1 Vocabulary and word knowledge

The purpose of this Section is to help your child learn a range of strategies to develop word knowledge and support word-finding skills. Learning new words in categories will extend vocabulary knowledge. Your child will learn category names and will understand that sub-groups exist within categories for items that share specific features, e.g., within the category of animals, some sub-groups are pets, wild, and farm animals. Other relationships between words will be taught such as opposites and synonyms. If useful, dictionary skills will be taught.

A specific format for **learning new words** will be devised in your child's vocabulary learning workbook. This will help your child develop a deeper understanding of all the features of each new word. Visual representations will be used as needed. The format will include recording the following aspects of word knowledge:

❖ the spelling and number of syllables
❖ a synonym and an antonym (similar and opposite words)
❖ specific features of each word which differentiate it from other words in the same category
❖ a sentence that uses the word
❖ a simple definition

Strategies for word-finding will be taught. Your child will learn about similarities and differences between items in the same category and will use these differences to differentiate his/her definitions of these words. Practice in giving a full and accurate definition of a word will focus on using the category name and at least one important semantic feature. For example, a full definition of the word 'knife' would include the category 'cutlery', and features such as its function, 'to cut up food' and its appearance, 'made of metal', 'sharp blade', etc. Your child will be encouraged to use descriptions such as these at times when he is experiencing a word-finding challenge. This helps the listener to understand what is meant, and it can provoke the word in the child's memory.

How you can help

Teaching in this Section will be tailored to meet your child's needs. Please provide information from your child's recent actual experiences of words that he needs support to understand. These may be derived from school topics or from your child's particular interests. Review the words added to the workbook and discuss all aspects of the word as it is set out. You can add new words as they arise, although if your child is learning about a particular topic in school or has a specific new hobby, new words can be added as a group. Once words are added to the book, it can be used as a reference to look through to help with revision. When your child is trying to think of the words he needs, you can support him to persist in finding the word he needs by asking one or more of the following questions:

* ❖ can you tell me what letter/sound the word begins with?
* ❖ can you describe the thing you are thinking of? (specific features)
* ❖ can you tell me what kind of thing it is? (category name)
* ❖ can you tell me what you use it for? (function)

SCIP Phase 2: LP 1

LP 1.1 Understanding semantic relationships between words

Activity 1: Understanding semantic categories

Purpose and target

To help the child understand how words and items can be grouped into categories.

Materials

Pictures from main familiar categories selected from, e.g., Winslow Press Color Library sets for clothes/food/transport/furniture/people/places.

Procedure

Explain the purpose of the task as putting things together that belong together in the same group.

Select two items and explain the reasons why they belong together, e.g., "The cow and the rabbit are both animals. The dog and cat are also animals so they can join them. This is a group called animals".

Ask the child to select another few items to join the group of animals. Model, saying, e.g., "The horse is also an animal", to repeat the category name.

Repeat with a few more categories, gradually allowing the child to select items to fit the category as he gains confidence with the task.

Continue to engage the child in forming and adding to groups as the activity proceeds and gradually introduce less familiar categories.

Once the child is confident, set out a mixed selection of pictures from two or three groups and ask the child to sort them. Encourage the child to name the item and the category.

Repeat and modify the level of complexity as required.

SCIP Phase 2: LP 1

LP 1.1 Understanding semantic relationships between words

Activity 2: Understanding relationships within categories

Purpose and target

To help the child understand that words and items in categories can be grouped into sub-categories.

Materials

Pictures from categories practised in LP 1.1 Activity 1.

Additional pictures of low frequency items from these same categories.

For example, animals – wild, farm, and pets; food – snacks, treats, junk, and healthy foods; clothes – outdoor, indoor, summer, and winter; vehicles – motorised, land, air, and water vehicles.

Pictures of new, less familiar categories.

Procedure

Use a category practised in Activity 1 and explain that there are lots of other groups within that category, e.g., "Last week we worked on putting pictures into groups. We put lots of animals together. Today, we are going to sort the animals into groups. We are going to find farm animals and wild animals".

Put two items together to form a sub-category and explain the reasons why they belong together, e.g., the cow and the rabbit are both animals that usually live on a farm. The chicken also lives on the farm so it can join them. This group is called farm animals.

Repeat using three wild animals to model the differences between the sub-categories.

Repeat with a few more categories gradually allowing the child to add items to the group as he gains confidence with the task.

Using one category at a time, set out some pictures from the categories just practised and ask the child to group the items. Support the child to explain his reasons and to name the categories created.

Repeat and modify the level of complexity as required.

SCIP Phase 2: LP 1

LP 1.1 Understanding semantic relationships between words

Activity 3: Understanding salient features of objects

Purpose and target

To help the child to understand that items in categories can be differentiated based on the salient features of each item (similarities and differences).

Materials

Pictures of high and low frequency items selected from, e.g., Winslow Press Color Library sets for clothes/food/transport/furniture/people/places.

Procedure

Set out up to ten items from one category only and explain that even though they are all from the same category it is possible to sort these items into smaller groups.

Present one picture and highlight the specific features that separate it from other members of the same category, e.g., transport: A car has four wheels, windscreen wipers, seats for four or five people.

Present a contrast item from the same group and point out the similarities and differences between the two items.

Focus on what is different between the two vehicles and use a key phrase that can help the child define the low frequency item, e.g., bus: It's like a car, but has seats for more people, lots of people travel in it, you pay to get on it, etc.

Repeat with another pair within this category and pairs from other categories and continue to model how to find the similarities and differences until the child is ready to reverse roles.

Role-reversal

Start by using the category items just discussed and ask the child to find two items that are alike but not exactly the same.

If necessary, offer two high frequency words.

Ask the child to explain the similarities and differences and repeat with a few other examples from this category to establish the child in this role.

Present a set of pictures in a new category and ask the child to find the similarities and differences between any two items, supporting as needed.

Gradually extend until you are using low frequency words and the child is able to consider the similarities and differences of unfamiliar items.

If school staff provide vocabulary related to school topics these can be incorporated into the activity.

Record some examples and key phrases to talk about definitions in the child's vocabulary workbook and make note of words the child needs to revise.

SCIP Phase 2: LP 1

LP 1.1 Understanding semantic relationships between words

Activity 4: Understanding functions of objects

Purpose and target

To help the child to understand that items in categories can be differentiated based on the function each item performs.

Materials

Pictures of high and low frequency items selected from, e.g., Winslow Press Color Library sets for clothes/food/transport/furniture/people/places/tools/utensils.

Procedure

Using a set of pictures from one category, e.g., tools or household items, explain that as well as knowing the category name, that it is important to know what each item is used for and what it does.

Present one picture and describe its functions. Highlight the specific functions that separate it from other members of the same category, e.g., we use a lamp to see better at home.

Present a contrast item and point out the similarities and differences, e.g., torch.

Focus on what is different between the two items and use a key phrase that can help the child define the low frequency item, e.g., It's like a lamp, but you can carry it around to help you see in the dark; you can take it outside and it will still work, it needs batteries to work, etc.

Repeat with another pair and continue to model with at least five pairs.

Role-reversal

Start by using the category items just discussed and ask the child to find two items that are alike in how the items are commonly used but are not exactly the same.

If necessary, offer two high frequency words.

Ask the child to explain the similarities and differences and repeat with a few other examples from this category to establish the child in this role.

Present a set of pictures in a new category and ask the child to find the similarities and differences in how items function between any two items, supporting as needed.

Gradually extend until you are using low frequency words and the child is able to consider functions of unfamiliar items.

If school staff provide vocabulary related to school topics these can be incorporated into the activity.

Record some examples and key phrases to talk about similarities and differences in the child's vocabulary workbook and make note of words the child needs to revise.

SCIP Phase 2: LP 1

LP 1.1 Understanding semantic relationships between words

Activity 5: Understanding definitions

Purpose and target

To help the child to understand that category names, functions, and specific semantic features are the essential elements of accurate word definitions.

Materials

Range of pictures of high and low frequency items selected from, e.g., Winslow Press Color Library sets.

Chart using symbols or written words showing three columns for category name, function, and specific feature.

Procedure

Explain that this work is learning how to give 'full' definitions using three pieces of information: Category name, function, and specific features. Use vocabulary relevant to the child.

Place up to ten cards face up on the table, including at least two from the same category, two with shared features, and two with shared functions.

Model a clear definition of an item using category, function, and feature.

Ask the child to 'work out' the one you have described.

When he selects it, explain that he could work it out because you told him all three things about it.

Put a tick against all three pieces of information on the chart.

Meta-challenge

Repeat for another item but only give one piece of information which does not differentiate it from the others.

Explain that he couldn't work it out because you told him only one thing.

Model how to give a complete definition with another four items.

Role-reversal

Using the same pictures, ask the child to define one item for you to work out. Use the chart to reinforce this.

When the child gives the definition, give feedback on the quality of the definition before 'working out' the answer, e.g., "I know that one, because you told me the category name, what you use it for and what it looks like".

Repeat until the child is confidently providing all available information as a definition.

If school staff provide vocabulary related to school topics these can be incorporated into the activity.

Record some examples and key phrases to talk about similarities and differences in the child's vocabulary workbook and make note of words the child needs to revise.

SCIP Phase 2: LP 1

LP 1.2 Consolidation and self-cueing

Activity 1: Understanding word knowledge

Purpose and target

To assist the child to understand and use a word-learning framework to support development of word knowledge across categories.

Materials

Pictures from categories practised and understood in LP 1.1.

LP 1.2 Activity 1 Resource or suitable word-learning template.

Vocabulary workbook.

Glue stick and pens.

Pictures of words that have been recorded for further practice in previous LP 1.1 work.

Procedure

Label the vocabulary book with a suitable name to help the child understand its purpose and stick a copy of the template into the inside cover for reference. Explain that this work is to help the child learn and remember new words.

Select a category and items that the child knows well.

Demonstrate how to use the template by writing a word that the child knows well as the target word.

Ask the child to write the word on the top left of the template.

Discuss each element with the child as you add information about the word into the template.

Emphasise how the semantic elements combine to create a definition.

Complete the diagram by writing a sentence using the word. The child's ideas can be used.

When you have completed all the sections, review the template and talk about each of the sections.

Focus on teaching any aspect that the child is unfamiliar with.

Repeat with at least four more words, modelling and explaining each step as you complete it and engaging the child in completing as much as he can for each word.

Add each template to the workbook.

Role-reversal

When the child is ready, use a new set of words from previous work or from topic vocabulary lists from school and support him to complete the template.

Support with any features that the child does not know and make a note of these for homework or future intervention.

SCIP Phase 2: LP 1

Resource

LP 1.2 Consolidation and self-cueing

Activity 1 Resource: Understanding word knowledge

Use this template to show how the elements of category name, features, and functions combine to create a definition that is accurate and complete.

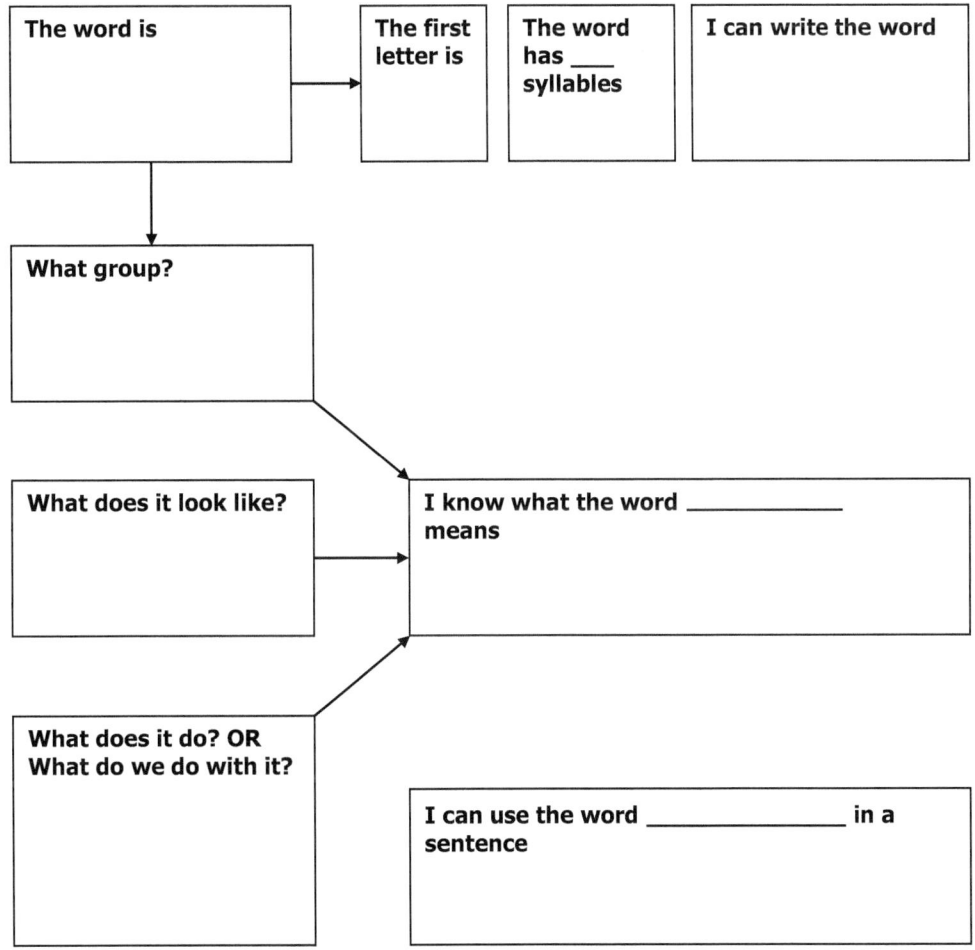

SCIP Phase 2: LP 1

LP 1.2 Consolidation and self-cueing

Activity 2: Consolidating understanding of word knowledge

Purpose and target

To consolidate the child's understanding that category names, functions, and specific
semantic features are the essential elements of accurate word definitions.

Materials

Broad selection of picture cards (nouns) in pairs from at least six different categories.

Picture of a star drawn on paper and measuring no more than the size of the picture cards
(this will be hidden under one picture in Game 2).

Procedure

Game 1: Password game

Give the child a set of six pictures from at least two categories and keep a matching set for
yourself.

Select one picture and give the child a description of it using the category name, feature, and
function.

Ask the child to 'work out' (not guess) the password from your description (i.e., the password
is the name of the object in the picture).

The child collects the pictures he has correctly worked out.

Keep the pictures the child has not worked out for a second try and give easier clues.

Use **role-reversal** when the child understands the game.

Use **meta-challenge** when the child has understood the game and can identify the missing
information in your clue.

Game 2: Find the star

Place up to 20 pictures face up on the desk from at least three different categories.

Ask the child to hide a star under one of the pictures and hide your eyes.

Say, "I am going to work out where the star is by asking questions about the words".

Start by asking category questions, e.g., "Is it under an animal?".

Eliminate as many pictures as you can by asking questions at this level and explain to the
child why this is a good way to start.

When you have one category left in the game, ask questions about the salient features or
functions.

Explain how each of these questions helps you get closer to the star.

Find the star and emphasise how you found it by asking the right questions.

Repeat and use **role-reversal** when the child understands the game.

SCIP Phase 2: LP 1

LP 1.2 Consolidation and self-cueing

Activity 3: Supporting self-cueing in conversation

Purpose and target

To help the child to use word knowledge to self-cue in conversation.

Materials

Pictures to act as prompts for a conversation that will require the child to use high and low frequency words, e.g., birthday party, trip to the museum, etc.

Procedure

Explain that the task is to practise describing and explaining words if we forget them when we are talking with our friends and teachers.

Engage the child in conversation on a topic of sufficient complexity that the child will need to use low frequency vocabulary.

Observe and support use of description and explanation if word-finding behaviours occur.

Explain how helpful the description was to you and that you could work out what the child meant and keep the conversation going.

Meta-challenge

It may be difficult to stimulate word-finding behaviours in conversation, so meta-challenge can be used to demonstrate the effect of description.

Act as if you have forgotten a word when talking with the child.

Model using a definition to cue the child into the word you mean while in the conversation and discuss how this helped the conversation to keep going.

Repeat with a few more words to demonstrate how to use the definition to cue the listener in, or to find the required word.

Explain that if he forgets a word, he can use these strategies to remember it or help the listener know what he means.

In other work, draw the child's attention to successful self-cueing strategies used.

SCIP Phase 2: LP 1

LP 1.3 Vocabulary enrichment

Activity 1: Understanding synonyms

Purpose and target

To help the child understand that synonyms are two different words with similar meanings and to be able to use synonyms in speech and writing.

Materials

LP 1.3 Activity 1 Resource.

Pen and paper.

Child's reading book or similar level texts.

Dictionary and thesaurus if needed.

Procedure

Explain that synonyms are two different words with similar meanings and that synonyms are used to make speaking, reading, and writing more interesting.

Use examples from the Activity Resource to demonstrate how to use two different words in the same sentence without changing the meaning.

Look the words up in the dictionary or thesaurus if needed and show how they are related.

Repeat using a few more examples until the child understands the task.

Personalisation

Open the child's reading book and select a sentence that could be changed by a synonym.

Write it out and choose a word that can be changed while keeping the same meaning.

Use the dictionary or thesaurus as needed.

Write out the new sentence and underline the synonyms.

Below this, write a sentence explaining that these two words are synonyms, e.g., rock and stone are synonyms; they have almost the same meaning.

Repeat with several examples until the child knows the word synonym and its meaning.

Engage the child in conversation about their interests (from ISCP).

Relay possible synonyms to the child for words they use in this conversation.

If needed, engage the child in writing a description of a suitable picture or the room you are in. If needed, write the description to the child's dictation.

At the end, review it together and change some words using synonyms.

For older children, explain that synonyms help add to the style, mood, atmosphere, and emotion of writing/talking.

SCIP Phase 2: LP 1

Resource

LP 1.3 Vocabulary enrichment

Activity 1 Resource: Understanding synonyms

Draw two boys talking to each other.

Say, "Look at this picture. I could say, Peter is *talking* to his brother, or I could say that Peter is *speaking* to his brother. Both are true. The words talking and speaking are synonyms. That means that they mean the same thing. We can change the words and the meaning stays the same".

Peter is <u>talking</u> to his brother. I could say, Peter is _____ to his brother.

Elephants are <u>huge</u>. I could say, elephants are _____.

I like to go to the <u>beach</u>. I could say, I like to go to the _____.

My sister is really <u>beautiful</u>. I could say, my sister is really _____.

Please close the door; it's <u>cold</u> in here. I could say, please close the door; it's _____ in here.

I lost my glasses and had to <u>look</u> everywhere for them. I could say, I lost my glasses and had to _____ everywhere for them.

Joanne is a <u>fast</u> runner. I could say, Joanne is a _____ runner.

My friend Jade <u>broke</u> a window. I could say, my friend Jade _____ a window.

Mum made a <u>nice</u> cake for my birthday. I could say, Mum made a _____ cake for my birthday.

I felt <u>happy</u> when I won the prize at the gala. I could say, I felt _____ when I won the prize at the gala.

SCIP Phase 2: LP 1

LP 1.3 Vocabulary enrichment

Activity 2: Understanding antonyms

Purpose and target

To help the child understand that antonyms are two words with opposite meanings and to be able to use antonyms in speech and writing.

Materials

LP 1.3 Activity 2 Resource.

Pen and paper.

Child's reading book or similar level texts.

Dictionary of opposites.

Procedure

Explain that antonyms are words with opposite meanings and that using antonyms changes the meaning of the sentence.

Use one example from the Activity Resource to demonstrate how to use different words in the same sentence to change the meaning.

Look the words up in the dictionary or thesaurus if appropriate and show how they are related.

Repeat using a few more examples until the child understands the task.

Personalisation

Open the child's reading book and select a sentence that could be changed by an antonym.

Write it out and underline the word that can be changed to change the meaning.

Use the dictionary or thesaurus as appropriate.

Write out the new sentence and underline the antonyms.

Below this, write a sentence explaining that these two words are antonyms, e.g., hot and cold are antonyms; they have opposite meaning.

Repeat with several examples until the child knows the word antonym and its meaning.

Engage the child in conversation about their interests (from ISCP).

Suggest possible antonyms to the child for words they use in this conversation, make this fun, e.g., "you *hate* playing football".

SCIP Phase 2: LP 1

Resource

LP 1.3 Vocabulary enrichment

Activity 2 Resource: Understanding antonyms

Draw two faces, one happy and one sad.

Say, "Look at these pictures, this face is <u>happy</u> and this face is <u>sad.</u> Happy and sad have opposite meanings, this means they are antonyms. Antonyms can change the meaning of the story. John was <u>happy</u> to go to school. John was <u>sad</u> to go to school. The meaning is not the same".

Fill the bucket with <u>dirty</u> water.
To change the meaning to the opposite, I can say, fill the bucket with _____ water.
Dirty and clean are antonyms.
Sally wanted a <u>big</u> piece of cake.
To change the meaning to the opposite, I can say, Sally wanted a _____ piece of
    cake.
It is <u>sunny</u> outside.
To change the meaning to the opposite, I can say, it is _____ outside.
I <u>love</u> broccoli and carrots.
To change the meaning to the opposite, I can say, I _____ broccoli and carrots.
Can you <u>open</u> the window please?
To change the meaning to the opposite, I can say, can you _____ the window please?
The fruit bowl was <u>full.</u>
To change the meaning to the opposite, I can say, the fruit bowl was _____.
Jason jumped over a <u>high</u> fence.
To change the meaning to the opposite, I can say, Jason jumped over a _____ fence.
Louise cooked a <u>delicious</u> meal for her friends.
To change the meaning to the opposite, I can say, Louise cooked a _____ meal
    for her friends.
Janice bought a <u>beautiful</u> dress at the shop on Saturday.
To change the meaning to the opposite, I can say, Janice bought a _____ dress at
    the shop on Saturday.
I don't want to go in that <u>old</u> house; it's too <u>dark.</u>
To change the meaning to the opposite, I can say, I don't want to go in that _____ house;
    it's too _____.

SCIP Phase 2: LP 1

LP 1.3 Vocabulary enrichment

Activity 3: Dictionary skills

Purpose and target

To assist the child in understanding the steps to follow in looking up words in a dictionary.

Materials

A dictionary matched to the child's ability.

List of words to look up in the dictionary.

LP 1.3 Activity 3 Resource or other suitable chart with step-by-step instructions.

Procedure

Explain the function and features of the chosen dictionary.

Explain how the pages are arranged with words in alphabetical order and that the two words at the very top of the page are the first and last words on this page. Explain how this helps us to find a word.

Show the child the checklist in the Activity Resource.

Model finding a word that the child knows while emphasising each step as you go through the process and ticking the column marked 'Done' before moving to the next step.

When you find the word, write the word and definition in the child's vocabulary workbook.

Repeat until the child is clear about the task.

Role-reversal

Assist the child to look up words he knows before looking for words he doesn't know.

SCIP Phase 2: LP 1

Resource

LP 1.3 Vocabulary enrichment

Activity 3 Resource: Dictionary skills

As each step is completed mark it off in the column marked 'Done' to help the child slow down and complete each step in order.

Step	What to do	Done
1	Open the dictionary at the section for words beginning with the first letter of the word you are checking. If possible, find the section for the first two letters.	
2	Read the words at the top of each page: these words are the first and last words on each page.	
3	Decide whether your word comes between the first word and last word or not. **If yes, your word will be on this page.** **If no, move to the next page and check the first and last words.** Keep moving through until you are on the right page.	
Tip: On a double page, you can check the first word on the left-hand page and the last word on the right-hand page to increase speed.		
4	When you are on the right page, decide if your word is closer to the first word or the last word and start looking in that place.	
5	Read each word and compare it to your word.	
6	When you find your word, check whether the word is listed as (N) for noun or (V) for verb and read the one that matches the sentence you are checking.	
7	There may be more than one entry for the word you are checking. Read all the entries until you find the one that matches the meaning in the sentence you are checking.	

Worked example: Looking up the word *fall*

Find the section for words beginning with 'f'.

Read the words at the top of each page: these words are the first and last words on each page.

fall is on the page where the first word is **fair** and the last word is **fall**.

Note that there are two separate entries for *fall* as a verb and as a noun.

Under *fall (verb)* there are 7 possible definitions.

Under *fall (noun)* there are 3 possible definitions.

Check each entry for the definition that best matches the sentence you are checking.

LP 2 Intervention content table

LP 2 Narrative construction

LP 2 Information

LP 2.1 Understanding inferences in picture sequences

1 Using relevant detail to make inferences

2 Explaining inferences in complex sequences

LP 2.2 Telling complex and personalised stories

1 Telling complex stories

2 Summarising stories

3 Telling stories from experiences

4 Telling recent events

LP 2.3 Constructing novel stories with plot

1 Introduction to creating new stories

2 Understanding character in stories

3 Understanding location in stories

4 Understanding fantasy and reality in stories

5 Creating novel stories

SCIP Phase 2: LP 2

Information

LP 2 Narrative construction

The purpose of this Section is to help your child learn a range of strategies to develop narrative storytelling skills. This Section makes use of traditional fairy tales, sets of sequence pictures of familiar events, school reading books, and stories of interest to your child to develop an understanding of how stories are created. Initially, your child will be taught how to find and use relevant detail in picture sequences to make inferences and predictions about other events in that story. As this skill develops, your child will be supported to order up to eight pictures into a coherent sequence.

A specific format or a 'story chart' for learning how narratives are constructed will be devised in your child's workbook. This will help your child develop a deeper understanding of all the features needed in stories. Photographs, drawings, and other visual representations will be used as needed. The format will include recording the following aspects of narrative construction:

❖ creating an introduction and setting the scene
❖ characters
❖ locations
❖ events
❖ feelings
❖ problems
❖ resolutions and conclusions

Work in this Section will enable your child to identify these elements in stories and to include them in his/her own narratives, gradually working towards telling events that have recently happened. Your child will receive explicit feedback on the quality of his/her narratives to help raise awareness of what he has and hasn't included, e.g., "You told me *who* was at the party, you didn't tell me *what happened*". Specific story elements are practised in depth such as how to add a new character, a new location, or a fantastical element to the story. As skill develops, your child will be invited to use their imagination to allow the opportunity to create completely novel stories.

How you can help

Teaching in this Section will be tailored to meet your child's needs. Please provide information from your child's familiar, recent experiences that will make suitable stories for retelling personal experiences. You will need to provide detail for each of the elements on your child's story chart. When talking to your child, you can give feedback on which elements he has told you and which you still need to know, e.g., "Can you tell me *where* this happened?".

SCIP Phase 2: LP 2

LP 2.1 Understanding inferences in picture sequences

Activity 1: Using relevant detail to make inferences

Purpose and target

To help the child to understand that details in picture sequences can be used to make inferences, predictions, and are needed for coherent narratives.

Materials

Winslow Press 6–8 step sequence sets.
Blank cards and sticky notes to draw inferred scenes, thoughts, words, or actions.
Arrow sticky notes to stick on the picture to highlight relevant details.

Procedure

Select two pictures from one sequence set where the inferences are easy to observe from details in the scenes, e.g., in the picture set, 'going to school' select the picture showing the forgotten bag on the doorstep with either the picture showing the child realising he has forgotten it or walking to school without the bag and not showing awareness of having left it.

Discuss this pair and focus on the details which help us work out how they are related.

Use the words 'inference' and 'make a prediction', e.g., his school bag is on the doorstep.

Ask the child to predict another event in the sequence.

Show the picture in the set that matches the prediction and continue to discuss the inferences.

Show another picture from the same set that is more open to interpretation, e.g., eating breakfast.

Discuss the inferences that can be made and ask the child where it is placed in the sequence, i.e., before leaving for school.

Repeat with another two pictures from this set, agreeing the order as you go.

When the sequence is complete tell the story, explaining the inferences from each picture and how each picture relates to the previous one as you go.

Emphasise and explain what world knowledge is – i.e., "it always happens like this" information.

Emphasise and explain what is implied in the picture, giving meaning to specific detail.

Ask questions such as "What happened that we didn't see?".

Draw scenes that are implied or not shown on blank cards, e.g., draw Mum driving back home, collecting the bag, and driving back to school.

Repeat with other sets adjusting the complexity and familiarity of the materials so that the child can understand the inferences from his own perspective and experience.

Gradually ask the child to add more detail independently.

Using more ambiguous pictures, e.g., "Are they putting the tent up or taking it down?", "Are they arriving or leaving?", can show that more information is needed before a decision can be made.

SCIP Phase 2: LP 2

LP 2.1 Understanding inferences in picture sequences

Activity 2: Explaining inferences in complex sequences

Purpose and target

To enable the child to make inferences from relevant detail in picture sequences and to use this information to create coherent narratives.

Materials

Winslow Press 4 step and 6–8 step sequence sets.

Blank cards and sticky notes to draw inferred scenes, thoughts, words, or actions.

Arrow sticky notes to stick on the picture to highlight relevant details.

Procedure

Continuing from Activity 1, explain that the task is to put as much of the story together with only some of the cards and to work out what information is missing.

Start with a 4-step picture sequence to demonstrate the task.

Set out two cards, discuss inferences, and make predictions as in Activity 1 and then show that your working out was correct by showing the remaining two pictures.

Role-reversal

Give the child some pictures from the set. Alternate the position in the sequence of the retained cards to reflect easy or harder inferences and predictions.

Support the child as required to set out the sequence and decide the position of the missing card(s).

Discuss and emphasise the relation between details and inferences as in Activity 1.

Support the child as required to work out what is on the retained card(s), e.g., by drawing some part of the missing events.

Show the retained card and discuss to support the child's reasoning.

Draw explicit attention to key inferences from the pictures and world knowledge.

SCIP Phase 2: LP 2

LP 2.2 Telling complex and personalised stories

Activity 1: Telling complex stories

Purpose and target

To help the child to further develop the ability to relate events and stories, listing key elements of the story from the following: Introduction, setting the scene, locations, characters, events, problems, feelings, resolutions, and conclusions.

Materials

Winslow Press 4 step and 6–8 step sequence sets.

Traditional stories in sequenced picture sets.

Blank cards to draw inferred scenes, thoughts, words, or actions.

Storytelling chart of symbols for each story element listed above, e.g., Black Sheep Press Narrative Resources or a checklist of 'wh–' questions for main elements.

Procedure

Create or adapt a chart of story elements appropriate for the child's ability and using words or symbols as needed.

Explain that the task is to tell a story and use the chart as a guide to make sure we tell all the 'important ideas'.

Model telling a story from a familiar sequence and mark off story elements on the chart as you go.

Repeat the same story and this time ask the child to listen and mark off the elements as you tell it.

Repeat with new stories and pictures until the child is familiar with the elements on the chart and can recognise the story elements in your narrative with some independence.

Role-reversal

Using a story that you have just told, ask the child to tell it in his own words.

As the child tells the story, mark off the elements on the chart. This will help the child keep track of what else he needs to explain.

Review each story and give explicit feedback on what has been achieved, e.g., "You told me who is in the story and what happened, but you didn't tell me where they were", etc.

Repeat with stories the child knows well and with harder and longer sequences until he is including sufficient detail.

Note which elements the child needs support with.

Note any changes in the child's sentence construction as narrative demands increase.

Record the chart and some examples of stories in the child's workbook.

Meta-challenge

Tell a story with missing elements and ask the child to identify which elements were left out and provide them to make the story complete.

SCIP Phase 2: LP 2

LP 2.2 Telling complex and personalised stories

Activity 2: Summarising stories

Purpose and target

To help the child to further develop the ability to retell events and stories, listing key aspects of the story from the following elements: Introduction, setting the scene, locations, characters, events, problems, feelings, resolutions, and conclusions.

Materials

Child's school reading book and other age-appropriate story books.

Traditional story book, e.g., Little Red Riding Hood.

Storytelling chart of symbols created in LP 2.2 Activity 1.

Blank cards to draw the story if necessary.

Procedure

Using the story chart created in Activity 1, explain that the task is to retell a story from a book and to use the chart as a guide to make sure we tell all the 'important ideas'.

Model telling a story from a familiar story book and mark each element off on the chart as you talk.

Role-reversal

Ask the child to retell the story from his reading book.

Mark off the elements on the chart as he is talking, with support as needed.

Review each story and give explicit feedback on what has been achieved, e.g., "You told me who is in the story and what happened, but you didn't tell me where they were", etc.

Repeat with other reading books or story books until the child can retell the story with some independence.

Meta-challenge

Tell a story with missing elements and ask the child to identify which elements were left out and provide them to make the story complete.

SCIP Phase 2: LP 2

LP 2.2 Telling complex and personalised stories

Activity 3: Telling stories from experiences

Purpose and target

To practise retelling stories and events that might typically happen in children's lives.

Materials

Scenes of childhood activities, such as days out at the park, the swimming pool, single pictures from sequencing sets showing suitable childhood activities, including pictures of shared adult/child experiences, e.g., cinema. Do not include challenging events.

Storytelling chart of symbols created in LP 2.2 Activity 1.

Blank cards and pens to draw additional detail for the story sequence.

Procedure

Explain that the task is to tell a story about things that a lot of children will have experienced.

Model telling a story using one of the pictures of typical childhood experiences that the child can relate to, e.g., cinema.

Draw simple pictures to expand on the main events and elements of the story that are not included in the stimulus picture.

Mark off on the story chart the elements you are telling as you go.

Role-reversal

Present another stimulus picture and support the child to imagine and tell the story while you mark off the elements on the story chart.

Review each story and give explicit feedback on what has been achieved, e.g., "You told me who is in the story and what happened, but you didn't tell me where they were", etc.

If the child starts to tell an event that has actually happened to him, support him to do this and draw some events to show his experience before moving on to Activity 4: Telling recent events.

Meta-challenge

Tell a story with missing elements and ask the child to identify which elements were left out and provide them to make the story complete.

Tell a story with a problem, e.g., the film is not showing at the cinema and discuss with the child how the people would feel and what they could do to make things better.

Record examples of stories in the child's workbook.

SCIP Phase 2: LP 2

LP 2.2 Telling complex and personalised stories
Activity 4: Telling recent events
Purpose and target

To practise retelling recent events that have happened with detail and in the expected sequence.

Materials

Ideas from the child's ISCP from parent and teacher report.
Storytelling chart created in LP 2.2 Activity 1.
Blank cards and pens to draw the story sequence.

Procedure

Use the story chart created in Activity 1 and explain that the task is to tell a story about something that has really happened to the child.

Model telling a story from your own recent experiences that the child can relate to, e.g., driving to school, morning routines, going to the cinema, etc.

Draw simple pictures to illustrate the main events and elements of the story.

Mark off on the chart the elements you are telling as you go.

Make the link explicit to the child that we can tell stories about ourselves and that we can include the important ideas to make it a full story.

Take an example from the ISCP and start to tell a story from the child's recent experience, e.g., "I know that on Saturday you went to the cinema".

Draw some pictures to get it started and then ask him to join in and take over telling the story as you draw out the events.

Support the child to start to tell the story while you mark off the elements on the chart

Review each story and give explicit feedback on what has been achieved, e.g., "You told me who is in the story and what happened, but you didn't tell me where they were", etc.

Repeat with other examples from yourself and from the child to model how to tell a complete story as required.

Record examples of stories in the child's workbook.

SCIP Phase 2: LP 2

LP 2.3 Constructing novel stories with plot
Activity 1: Introduction to creating new stories
Purpose and target

To support the child to create a simple novel story from given elements.

Materials

Mixed Up Fairy Tales book by Nick Sharratt or similar book.

Traditional tales prepared in sequenced sets.

Blank cards to add novel story events as suggested by the child.

Procedure

Explain the task as making up new stories using people and events already known.

Use the *Mixed Up Fairy Tales* book to show how people and events from one story can be mixed together to make new stories.

Show that some of these stories can be funny, impossible, or possible, e.g., Goldilocks could marry a handsome prince, but she couldn't marry a treasure chest.

Using the traditional tales sequenced pictures; model a short story using pictures from one story and one or two characters from another. For example, "Goldilocks is on her way to the house of the three bears, but on the way, she meets Little Red Riding Hood in the forest. What happens next?".

Draw ideas on the blank cards to complete the story.

Give the new story a title and add the child's name as author to the front cover if a book is created.

Repeat using the child's suggestions and favourite stories.

Aim for novelty, flexibility, and humour.

Repeat with a variety of starter stimuli, e.g., objects/pictures/people.

Repeat with other sequences relating to real events.

Gradually support the child to create the stories independently.

SCIP Phase 2: LP 2

LP 2.3 Constructing novel stories with plot

Activity 2: Understanding character in stories

Purpose and target

To help the child understand how to introduce a new character to a story and create a role for that character in the story.

Materials

Sequence pictures of traditional tales, Winslow Press sequence sets, or similar.

Cut out characters from well-known TV programmes or cartoons.

Blank cards to add novel story events as suggested by the child.

Procedure

Explain the task as learning how to bring new people into a story; introduce and explain them.

Using the traditional tales sequenced pictures, model a short story using pictures from one story.

Introduce an unexpected character, e.g., a cartoon character, at an appropriate point in the story.

Reflect with the child on what you said to introduce the new person, e.g., "When all of sudden, along came Harry Potter. Goldilocks was very surprised to see Harry Potter!" and so on.

Discuss with the child what the new person could do in the story and how that character can influence events.

Draw out the story and discuss positive and negative consequences for the story and characters.

Draw ideas on the blank cards to complete the story.

Give the new story a title and add the child's name as author to the front cover if making a book.

Repeat using the child's suggestions and favourite stories and characters.

Write down some of the ways you can introduce a new character.

Aim for novelty, flexibility, and humour, but ensure that the child understands this as a creative activity.

Gradually support the child to create the stories independently.

Note: For children whose needs include mixing fantasy and reality elements in narratives, this activity may be completed alongside LP 2 Activity 4: Understanding fantasy and reality in stories.

SCIP Phase 2: LP 2

LP 2.3 Constructing novel stories with plot

Activity 3: Understanding location in stories

Purpose and target

To help the child understand how to introduce a change of location to a story and to make this meaningful in the story.

Materials

Sequence pictures of traditional tales, Winslow Press sequence sets, or similar.

Pictures or drawings of a variety of different locations.

Blank cards to add novel story events as suggested by the child.

Procedure

Explain the task as learning how to introduce and explain a change of location in a story.

Using the traditional tales sequenced pictures, model a short story using pictures from one story.

Introduce the new location at an appropriate point in the story.

Reflect with the child on what you said to introduce the new place, e.g., say, "On the way to Grandma's house, Little Red Riding Hood went to play on the swings. She liked going to the park. When she was in the park, she ...", etc.

Discuss with the child what the person could do in the story now she/he is in the new place and how this influences events.

Draw out the story and discuss positive and negative consequences of the change in location.

Draw ideas on the blank cards to complete the story.

Give the new story a title and add the child's name as author to the front cover if making a book.

Repeat using the child's suggestions and favourite stories and characters that he likes.

Write down some of the ways you can introduce a new location.

Aim for novelty, flexibility, and humour.

Gradually support the child to create the stories independently.

SCIP Phase 2: LP 2

LP 2.3 Constructing novel stories with plot

Activity 4: Understanding fantasy and reality in stories

Purpose and target

To help the child understand how to introduce a fantasy element into a story and to make this meaningful in the story.

Materials

Winslow Press 6–8 sequence sets or similar.

Pictures or drawings of a variety of different magical creatures: Fairy godmother, Harry Potter, witch, wizard, magician, etc. according to child's age/preferences.

Blank cards to add novel story events as suggested by the child.

Procedure

Explain the task as learning how to introduce and use fantasy in a story.

Using one sequenced set of pictures of everyday events, tell a short story without a fantasy element.

Repeat and introduce the magical element at a chosen point in the story.

Reflect with the child on what you said to introduce the magical event, e.g., "James was on his way to school. It was Sports Day, and he was very excited. He started thinking about winning the running race. Suddenly, a wizard popped up in front of his eyes! James said ...", etc.

Discuss with the child what the magic person could do in the story and how this influences events.

Draw out the story and discuss consequences of the magical element.

Draw ideas on the blank cards to complete the story.

Give the new story a title and add the child's name as author to the front cover if making a book.

Repeat using the child's suggestions and favourite stories and magical characters.

Write down some of the ways you can introduce a new magical character.

Aim for novelty, flexibility, and humour.

Gradually support the child to create the stories independently.

Personalisation

If the child often mixes fantasy and reality in his own conversation and narratives, use examples from the child's ISCP of how he does this and use this as an opportunity to reflect on the child's use of fantasy and reality in conversation.

Use alongside ideas from PRAG 5.3 Activity 1: Identifying mismatches and solutions in style, if this is an area of need for the child.

SCIP Phase 2: LP 2

LP 2.3 Constructing novel stories with plot

Activity 5: Creating novel stories

Purpose and target

To practise creating novel stories from given ideas or from the child's own imagination that draws on the structure of stories taught in this Section.

Materials

Black Sheep Press Speaking and Listening Pack scenes and characters (or similar).

Selection of characters, locations, and events from previous activities.

Blank cards to illustrate novel story events as suggested by the child.

Procedure

Explain the task as learning how to create new stories.

Show the child a selection of prepared scenes and characters.

Select a scene and a character and set the scene in a typical way and write this down, e.g., 'One sunny day, Luke was playing in the garden'.

Explain that you now need to decide what could happen from your imagination, e.g., "I can make up what happens next using my imagination".

Introduce characters, actions, and events to make a new simple story.

Draw each event and character on the blank cards to complete each step in the story.

Aim for a story that is possible, i.e., not a fantasy story.

Model a few stories and engage the child in adding ideas as you work.

Role-reversal

Ask the child to choose a different scene and character to tell a new story.

Support as needed to create a coherent story.

Draw the story on the blank cards as the child narrates.

Give the new story a title and add the child's name as author to the front cover if making a
book.
Repeat until the child is showing some independence.

Meta-challenge

Tell a story with missing elements and ask the child to identify which elements were left out
and provide them to make the story complete.

LP 3 Intervention content table

SCIP Phase 2	LP 3 Intervention content table

LP 3 Non-literal language

LP 3 Information

LP 3.1 Understanding homophones

1 Understanding multiple meanings for words

2 Understanding homophones in jokes plus Resource

3 Understanding homophones in text plus Resource

LP 3.2 Understanding literal and non-literal meanings

1 Understanding idioms

2 Using idioms

LP 3.3 Understanding non-literal meanings in context

1 Understanding idioms in social contexts

2 Understanding idioms in recent events (personalised)

SCIP Phase 2: LP 3

Information

LP 3 Non-literal language

The purpose of this Section is to help your child understand the ways that words or phrases can be used non-literally to mean something other than the literal meaning of the words. The Section starts by teaching homophones. Homophones are words that sound the same but have two or more different meanings. This introduces the idea that sometimes we need to check the meaning of words in a particular context. The homophones are taught as pairs of words before then being used in sentences so that the meaning can be worked out from the rest of the sentence (the meaning in context). Homophones can be used in jokes, and this Section includes teaching on how to work out the two meanings for the homophone in a joke and to predict what the punchline might be. Building on this idea of multiple meanings sets the scene for working on idioms and other non-literal expressions. Your child will be taught a set of idioms and their non-literal meanings. Your child will be taught to check meanings when unsure and to use the context (written words or social situation) to work out which meaning is intended.

Throughout this Section, the emphasis is on your child being able to identify idioms and homophones and to ask for explanation if he is confused. A book of homophones and idioms will be compiled as work is completed.

How you can help

Teaching in this Section can be tailored to meet your child's needs. Please provide information from your child's recent actual experiences when he has found it challenging to understand a speaker's intended meaning. Once the workbooks have been started, you can add new idioms or homophones as they arise in conversation using the format provided.

SCIP Phase 2: LP 3

LP 3.1 Understanding homophones

Activity 1: Understanding multiple meanings for words

Purpose and target

To help the child understand that homophones are words with more than one meaning but which sound the same.

Materials

A small workbook specifically for learning homophones and named My Book of Homophones.

Fun Deck Multiple Meanings or lists of homophones with matching pictures to illustrate both meanings.

Procedure

Explain the task as understanding that sometimes a word can have two meanings.

Using a homophone for which the child will already know both meanings, write the word on both facing pages in the homophones workbook, e.g., bat is a *homophone*, it means a little animal and it means something to hit a ball with.

Add sentences and draw a picture to illustrate meanings if useful.

Repeat with another familiar word until the child is sure of the task.

Repeat with other sets, asking the child to contribute his ideas on the meanings and scaffold his responses to teach both meanings.

Keep adding words and pictures to the workbook as this task is completed.

SCIP Phase 2: LP 3

LP 3.1 Understanding homophones

Activity 2: Understanding homophones in jokes

Purpose and target

To develop the child's understanding that homophones can be used to tell jokes.

Materials

Age-appropriate joke book or jokes from the Activity Resource 2.

Different coloured pens.

Thought bubble sticky notes.

Procedure

Following Activity 1, explain the task as understanding that homophones can be used in jokes to make us laugh

Select one joke from the Activity Resource and write out the joke in full and highlight the homophone.

Explain how one part of the joke makes us think of one of the meanings and another part of the joke makes us think of the other meaning of the homophone.

Draw two thinking bubbles below the joke and label them 'meaning 1' and 'meaning 2'.

Write the meanings of the homophone inside these thinking bubbles, emphasising the two meanings for the same word.

Using different coloured pens, show the child that the words in one part of the joke relate to 'meaning 1' and that other words in the joke make us think of 'meaning 2'.

Explain that the joke works because we keep thinking about 'meaning 1' for the whole joke even though in another part, usually the punchline, the words make us think of 'meaning 2'.

Use this explicit step-by-step approach to work through a few jokes which use homophones the child knows until he understands how to detect the homophone and why it is funny.

When the child understands the task, present a new joke and engage him in working out the possible answers based on the homophone.

Record some examples in the child's workbook and suggest some jokes the child can learn to tell family and friends.

Using jokes that have the homophone in the question part of the joke, not the punchline, may be harder to work out and may require more explanation.

SCIP Phase 2: LP 3

Resource

LP 3.1 Understanding homophones

Activity 2 Resource: Understanding homophones in jokes

What building has the most stories?
The library.

What can you find in the middle of Paris?
The letter R.

What's black and white and red all over?
A newspaper.

Why was the baby ant confused?
All his uncles were ants!

What makes an octopus laugh?
Ten tickles.

What is a moth's favourite subject in school?
Mothematics.

Why don't bikes stand up by themselves?
They are too tired.

Why don't African animals play games?
There are too many cheetahs.

What do skeletons use to speak to their friends?
A mobile bone.

What can run but never walks, has a mouth but never talks, has a head but never weeps, and has a bed but never sleeps?
A river.

Teacher: Ben, be careful your purse is open. Someone might take your money!
Ben: Oh, no. I left it open so I can get more money.
Teacher: How can you get more money?
Ben: The weather report said we would have some change in our weather!

SCIP Phase 2: LP 3

LP 3.1 Understanding homophones

Activity 3: Understanding homophones in text

Purpose and target

To help the child understand that the meaning of homophones in stories and texts is related to the context provided.

Materials

Short paragraphs based on homophones practised in Activity 1.
Thought bubble sticky notes.
Homophone poem in Activity Resource 3

Procedure

Explain the task as understanding that sometimes homophones are used in stories, and we need to understand the right meaning of the homophone for that story.

Using the homophones used in Activity 1, create short stories to illustrate that the meaning of the homophone is related to the rest of the story. For example, "The boy was looking for his bat. He looked under the bed and behind the wardrobe. [Up to here, bat could be either the animal or the sports equipment.] Mum said, 'Hurry up, Ben. You'll be late for cricket'".

Write out the story and write the two meanings of bat in two thinking bubbles as in Activity 2. As the story progresses, discuss how the meaning isn't clear; if it was a pet bat, it might have got out of its special cage and be hiding in a dark place. Explain how the ending helps us to be sure that the boy is looking for a cricket bat and not an animal.

Repeat with a few more examples until the child can identify a homophone in the story and understands how to look within the story for its meaning.

SCIP Phase 2: LP 3

Resource

LP 3.1 Understanding homophones

Activity 3 Resource: Understanding homophones in text

Have you ever seen? (Author unknown)

Have you ever seen a sheet on a riverbed?

Or a single hair on a hammer's head?

Does the needle ever wink its eye?

Why doesn't the wing of a building fly?

Can you tickle the ribs of a parasol?

Or open the trunk of a tree at all?

Are the teeth of a comb ever going to bite?

Have the hands of a clock any left, or right?

Can the garden plot be deep and dark?

And what is the sound of the oak tree's bark?

Has the foot of a mountain got a really big toe?

If you like homophones, then you will know!

SCIP Phase 2: LP 3

LP 3.2 Understanding literal and non-literal meanings

Activity 1: Understanding idioms

Purpose and target

To help the child understand that idioms are expressions that can be interpreted as a whole; and to demonstrate how to use requests for clarification in understanding idiomatic speech.

Materials

A small workbook specifically for learning idioms and named, e.g., My Book of Idioms.

Book – *120 Idioms at Your Fingertips*.

Black Sheep Press Speech Bubbles.

Book – *What Did You Say, What Do You Mean?* or similar.

Examples of idioms the child knows and doesn't know from parent and teacher report.

Procedure

Explain the task as understanding that sometimes people use 'sayings', 'idioms', or 'expressions' and that these expressions are a different way of saying what we mean.

Select an idiom the child knows to use as the worked example and write this idiom on one page of the workbook.

Draw a speech bubble and write the idiom inside and a thinking bubble and write the intended meaning inside.

Discuss thoroughly detailing the literal meaning and the non-literal meaning, using matched vocabulary to describe this difference.

Repeat with a few more familiar examples until the child understands the task.

Complete the book with a comprehensive set of idioms appropriate to the child's age.

Personalisation

Select some idioms that have been reported as problematic or confusing for the child.

Take each in turn and add them to the workbook as before.

Explain in detail the non-literal meaning and explain how each might be used with details of e.g., "So when Grandma says, 'Get your skates on', you will know that she wants you to hurry up".

Use role-play if needed to consolidate.

SCIP Phase 2: LP 3

LP 3.2 Understanding literal and non-literal meanings

Activity 2: Using idioms

Purpose and target

To consolidate idiom understanding and practise using chosen or personalised idioms.

Materials

Pictures to prompt recall of an idiom, e.g., sock for 'pull your socks up', a head for 'off the top of my head', skates for 'get your skates on', etc.

Paper clips and a magnetic fishing rod for a fishing game.

Procedure

Explain the task as practising using idioms.

Present up to ten pictures face down on the desk, each with a paper clip on it.

Use the fishing rod to start fishing for a picture and select one.

Turn it over and explain what one idiom for this picture could be. For example, "I've got a horse. One idiom could be 'hold your horses'".

Explain what the idiom means and who might say it, e.g., "That means slow down, and the teacher might say that if you were rushing your work".

Role-play how to use this idiom in an interaction if needed.

Take turns with the child in fishing for all the pictures.

Support the child to generate an idiom for each picture as needed.

Model the response and explanation in your turns.

Ensure the child understands the meanings and who would use the idiom and encourage the child to ask for help if he can't think of an idiom or the meaning.

Personalisation

Repeat the game using some idioms that have been reported as challenging for the child by parents, school staff, or from assessment.

Support the child to ask for help if he can't think of an idiom or the meaning.

SCIP Phase 2: LP 3

LP 3.3 Understanding non-literal meanings in context

Activity 1: Understanding idioms in social contexts

Purpose and target

To engage the child in recognising and understanding the social contexts where idioms are used.

Materials

Pictures of everyday social scenes relevant to child's experiences, selected from sequencing sets such as Schubi Tell Me About It sequences, Combimage cards, or similar.

Speech bubble sticky notes.

Scripts and idioms to match scenes.

Different coloured pens.

Procedure

Explain the task as working out who is using an idiom and why.

Set out one picture and describe the scene and events in detail as described in LP 2 activities.

Make and explain inferences about thoughts and intentions.

Add examples of what the characters might say in the speech bubbles.

Write one idiom in a speech bubble using different colour ink.

Discuss the literal and non-literal meanings for the idiom.

Explain what will happen if the literal meaning is taken, e.g., the boy will feel a bit confused.

Explain what the idiom means, what to do when you hear it and understand it, and what to do when you don't know it and don't understand.

Role-play to practise idioms if the child needs additional scaffolding to understand.

Meta-challenge

Set up a role-play with the child and explain the context, e.g., bowling, supermarket, etc.

Start a conversation and use an idiom that you have not already used and is not known by the child.

Observe and if the child does not understand that the phrase is an idiom, explain that he needs to ask for clarification.

Repeat with a few more unknown idioms until the child can confidently listen and ask, e.g. "What does shake a leg mean?".

SCIP Phase 2: LP 3

LP 3.3 Understanding non-literal meanings in context

Activity 2: Understanding idioms in recent events (personalised)

Purpose and target

To help the child understand when idioms and idiomatic language have been used in situations recently or regularly experienced and to use requests for clarification in understanding idiomatic speech.

Materials

List of problematic idioms from the child's ISCP.

List of idiomatic language used in class or collected in observation or from discussion with the teacher or parent.

Speech bubble and thought bubble sticky notes.

Different coloured pens.

Procedure

Explain the task as thinking about idioms that people use in school and at home so that the child can understand what they mean or can confidently ask for clarification.

Draw a picture to illustrate a recent or regular event where idioms are used and not understood.

Describe the scene and events in detail.

Make and explain inferences about the speaker's thoughts and intentions.

Add an idiom or idiomatic phrase to one of the speech bubbles using different coloured ink.

Discuss the idiom's literal and non-literal meanings.

Explain what happened, e.g., "Your teacher said, 'One step at a time'. She means, let's do this bit first, then the next bit. She doesn't mean get up and walk around, taking one step after the other. You were confused when she said, 'One step at a time'. It was an idiom. When you hear an idiom that you don't know, it's OK to ask for an explanation".

Draw a scene to match what probably happened – the child felt confused, did the wrong thing, the teacher said, "please sit down", "where are you going?", etc.

Explain what the idiom means and what to do when you hear it and understand, and what to do when you don't know it and don't understand.

Role-play to practise this idiom if needed to consolidate.

Repeat with examples of non-specific instructions if these have been observed as problematic, e.g., put it on the side.

Provide feedback to parent and teacher on idiomatic phrases practised for support in real life.

LP 4 Intervention content table

SCIP Phase 2	LP 4 Intervention content table

LP 4 Discourse comprehension

LP 4 Information

LP 4.1 Improving memory and listening

1 Developing memory strategies plus Resource

LP 4.2 Understanding verbal inferences

1 Understanding why-because inferences

2 Understanding inferences from words plus Resource

3 Working out word meaning from context plus Resource

4 Understanding inferences in short stories plus Resource

LP 4.3 Understanding stories

1 Understanding story maps

2 Predicting endings

3 Looking back for information

4 Making mental maps of stories

SCIP Phase 2: LP 4

Information

LP 4 Discourse comprehension

The purpose of this Section is to help your child learn a range of strategies to improve his/her ability to listen to and understand longer spoken instructions or information. This Section starts by teaching strategies to listen to longer and more complex verbal information such as repeating the instruction immediately after hearing it (rehearsal), saying it while completing the task (monitoring themselves and keeping their focus on the task), and holding the information in his/her head in 'chunks' and using fingers to count the 'chunks' off as they are completed.

As this skill develops, your child will be supported to use this skill while listening to stories of increasing length and complexity. Specific skills are taught as needed to enable your child to:

❖ understand 'why–because' reasoning and answer 'why' questions using the word 'because'
❖ identify words in text that he doesn't know and learn how to use the meaning of the sentence to work out the meaning of the unknown word
❖ listen actively to stories and be able to make inferences from spoken texts (no pictures)
❖ integrate information from oral stories and make predictions for how the story can end
❖ break down the story into its elements, such as characters, main events, purpose, problems, motivations, and resolutions
❖ build mental visual representations of stories to assist comprehension and to show how this helps comprehension
❖ use the strategy of looking back at the picture or text of a story to check information and answer questions

A degree of reading ability will be required for most stories and the stories used in this Section will be matched to your child's reading ability.

How you can help

Teaching in this Section will be tailored to meet your child's needs. Please provide information on your child's preferences for stories and suggest stories your child enjoys but for which some support for comprehension is needed. When reading with your child, you can give feedback as to whether he can remember the answers to the questions or whether he needs to re-read the story, i.e., 'look back' to check. Other strategies will be shared as your child completes this work.

SCIP Phase 2: LP 4

LP 4.1 Improving memory and listening

Activity 1: Developing memory strategies

Purpose and target

To encourage the child to use taught working memory strategies to listen to longer and more complex verbal information.

Materials

Composite pictures that contain a wide range of contrasting people, events, adjectives, nouns, and verbs, e.g., *You Choose* by Nick Sharratt and Pippa Goodhart or sets of single pictures as described in the Activity 1 Resource.

A4 Card to make a chart of memory strategies and stickers or stamps to act as rewards.

Procedure

Explain the task as learning how to remember what someone says by listening in a special way, i.e., by using three new strategies.

Model each of these three strategies: Counting the things to remember on our fingers (chunking); repeating the information aloud to keep it in our head (rehearsal); and saying it while we are doing the task (monitoring).

Write these on a chart or use a symbol to represent each strategy.

Show the child the composite picture and say, "I am going to show you how to remember what someone says. I am looking for a girl with a yellow t-shirt and a cat smiling. That's two things". Hold up two fingers and point to one finger at a time as you repeat the instruction in two 'chunks'.

Explain how this helps, by reminding you of the two things to look for.

Repeat the information aloud and explain how this helps you remember.

Now look at the picture and say the information aloud and hold up your fingers as you find the first thing and then the second.

Explain that these actions help because they help you to remember and keep thinking about the words as you look at all the interesting things on the picture. Explain that you don't forget or lose concentration.

Add a reward stamp under each symbol on the chart as you use it.

Start the child with an instruction using only single words and gradually increase the length following the order set out in the Activity Resource.

Emphasise each strategy every time and reflect to the child when they use it and why it helps.

Mark the child's use of the strategies on the chart for each attempt and give clear feedback. Say, "You could find all those things because you told yourself what to look for".

Find the level where the child needs to use the strategies to support recall and practise at this level.

Encourage asking for repetition and clarification.

Ensure that the vocabulary is well-known by the child so that this is not a barrier to completion and keep the verbal information within the child's ability until he can use the strategies of chunking, rehearsal, and monitoring without reminders.

Turn the picture over when giving the instruction and extend the length of time between giving the instruction and the child being able to see the picture and complete it.

SCIP Phase 2: LP 4
Resource

LP 4.1 Improving memory and listening
Activity 1 Resource: Developing memory strategies

This activity is designed to enable the child to develop strategies to listen to longer and more complex verbal information. The task aims to develop his skills in a stepwise fashion by providing the child with success at each level using the specified strategies before moving on to longer instructions.

As an alternative to composite pictures, or the *You Choose* book, create sets of the following:

- ❖ pictures of nouns that can be modified by an adjective and a range of pictures to represent adjectives (size, colour, quality)
- ❖ pictures of someone doing an action and a contrasting picture of the same action performed by a different person, e.g., man running, girl running

Lay out a set of contrasting nouns, verbs, and adjectives and noun plus verb pictures.

Create sets of phrases and clauses for each of the combinations in these picture sets, for example, Adj Adj N, Int Adj N, V Adv, Prep N, and SV, SVO, SVAdv*.

Deliver an instruction for the child to select from the array of pictures, e.g., a big green hat (Det Adj Adj N), running quickly in the park (V Adv Prep Det N), etc.

Increase the length of the verbal information in this order. All examples here are taken from *You Choose* by Nick Sharratt and Pippa Goodhart, pages 7–8.

Order	Construction	Example
1.	Single word level	Cooker, chair, and teddy bear
2.	Word + phrase	Cat on a chair
3.	Word + word + phrase	Clock and girl with black hair
4.	Phrase + phrase	Jug on the piano and a roaring fire
5.	Word + phrase + phrase	Cactus, sizzling sausages, and a stool beside a chest
6.	Clause + phrase	The cat is sitting on a chair and smiling at us
7.	Phrase + phrase + phrase	Old-fashioned record player, fish in a fountain, and a gnome with a fishing rod
8.	Phrase + phrase + clause	Blue fan on a desk, a doll's house, and a red pan is bubbling on the cooker
9.	Clause + clause + phrase	There are three sausages on the BBQ, a boy is holding a key, and a blue trampoline
10.	Clause + clause + clause	Humpty Dumpty is relaxing on the sofa, the candles are burning, and a train is running around a track

* Refer to grammatical categories. Adj = adjective (big), Adv = adverb (slowly), Det = determiner (the, a), Int = intensifier (very), O = object (ball), Prep = preposition (on), N = noun (grass, ball), S = subject (of the sentence, e.g., she), V = verb (walk).

SCIP Phase 2: LP 4

LP 4.2 Understanding verbal inferences

Activity 1: Understanding why–because inferences

Purpose and target

To help the child understand 'why–because' reasoning in pictures and answer why questions using the word 'because'.

Materials

Why–because cards from Super Duper Fun Decks or *Think It Say It* by Luanne Martin with a set of why questions for each picture.
Cards with the words or symbols for WHY? and BECAUSE.

Procedure

Explain the task as learning to ask 'why?' questions and give 'because' answers.
Select one picture and point to one part of it. Ask a 'why' question about this part of the picture. Repeat the question, e.g., "Why is the road wet?".
Model the answer, "The road is wet *because* it is raining". Emphasise the word 'because'.
Place the written or symbol cards in order, 'why' first, followed by 'because'.
Repeat the question and answer pointing to the two words/symbols on the cards.
Repeat with a new picture and questions until the child is confident of the task.
Ask for more than one reason within the material, e.g., why was the road wet = it had rained (obvious) or a burst water pipe (less obvious).

Role-reversal

Engage the child by suggesting some parts of the picture for him to create a 'why' question.
Support him to ask the 'why' question and give a model answer.
Work your way through the materials supporting the child to formulate some of the 'why' questions and provide answers using 'because'.

Meta-challenge

When the child is confidently asking and answering, you can give some answers with deliberate mistakes. Support the child to notice the mistakes and offer help to correct as needed.

SCIP Phase 2: LP 4

LP 4.2 Understanding verbal inferences

Activity 2: Understanding inferences from words

Purpose and target

To develop the child's understanding of inferences from simple verbal information when no visual context is provided.

Materials

LP 4.2 Activity 2 Resource.

Selection of character faces (no visual clues to context).

Winslow Press Verb Color cards, e.g., laughing, writing, cooking, or similar.

Procedure

Explain the task as learning to work things out by thinking about the words we know.

Select one character picture and explain, "We are going to work out some things about these people. For example, this man is a farmer. We cannot see anything other than his face, but we can work out that he lives on a farm. We know he will wear overalls because his job is messy. Overalls will keep his clothes clean", etc.

Explain how you know this. "Farmers always live on farms".

Repeat with another character, e.g., a nurse.

Repeat with other character pictures and support the child to think about what they may wear, look like, what they will say, who/what they might work with, etc.

Engage the child in providing more of the information as you proceed through this.

Write and draw word maps and images to support the child as required.

Next move on to inferences from verbs and encourage the child to use world knowledge and inference, e.g., "Why is the man writing? What might he write? Who is the letter for?".

Use more unfamiliar examples, e.g., brake lights suddenly come on in the car in front; whilst watching TV you hear scratching at the door.

Role-reversal

Ask the child to select a card for you to work out an inference and offer support to monitor your answers as needed.

Meta-challenge

When the child is confidently asking and reflecting on your answers, you can give some answers that are incorrect in some responses. Support the child to notice the deliberate mistakes and offer help to correct as needed.

SCIP Phase 2: LP 4

Resource

LP 4.2 Understanding verbal inferences

Activity 2 Resource: Understanding inferences from words

Using pictures of faces and a role or job to make inferences

Characters/roles	Questions to ask
This person is a doctor.	What does she/he look like?
This person is a singer.	Where will she/he work?
This person is a mechanic.	What will she/he say?
This person is a teacher.	What does she/he like to do?
This person is a computer operator.	What does she/he drive to work?
This person is a nurse.	Who does she/he work with?
This person is a policeman.	What equipment might she/he use at work?
This person is a vet.	What might make her/him happy?
This person serves food.	
This person is a builder.	
This person is a farmer.	
This person is an author.	

Actions and questions to ask	Using Verb Color Cards to infer context
This woman is putting on some sparkly earrings	**Why is the man cutting paper?**
Why is she doing this?	What might he be making?
Where could she be going?	Who might it be for?
What time is it?	What might he be thinking?
Who will she see?	What might he be feeling?
What might she say?	
This man is putting on a hat	**Why is the boy laughing?**
Why is he doing this?	Where might he be?
What could the weather be like?	How might he be feeling?
Where could he be going? Who might he see?	What might he say?
What might he do?	
This man is packing a suitcase	**Why is the girl pointing?**
Why is he doing this?	What might she be pointing at?
Where could he be going?	How might she be feeling?
Who might be going with him?	Who else might be there?
What time of year could it be?	What might she say?
What kind of clothes might he be packing?	What might someone else say?
This woman is buying wrapping paper	**Why is the man writing?**
Why is she doing this?	What might he be writing?
Where could she be? What time of year could it be?	Who is the list for? What might it say?
Whose present could it be?	What might he be thinking?
What might she be saying? How much might it cost?	Where might he take it?
This woman is writing a letter	**Why is the girl cooking?**
Why is she doing this?	Who is it for?
Who could she be writing to?	How might she be feeling?
What might she be saying? Where could she be?	What might she be thinking?
	Who else might be there?
	What might she say?

SCIP Phase 2: LP 4

LP 4.2 Understanding verbal inferences

Activity 3: Working out word meaning from context

Purpose and target

To help the child learn how to identify words in text that he doesn't know and how to use the meaning of the sentence to work out the meaning of the unknown word.

Materials

LP 4.2 Activity 3 Resource

Sentences with nonsense words embedded in such a way as to be able to determine their meaning.

Scripts with real words that the child does not know but can work out from the meaning of the sentence(s).

Procedure

Explain the task as learning to work things out by thinking about the words we know. Explain that there are two steps. Step 1, 'find the word I don't know'. Step 2, 'work out the meaning from the rest of the sentence'.

Select one sentence and read it aloud. Point out the nonsense word and explain what this is, and that it is possible to work out what it means by looking at the rest of the sentence.

Explain how you know this, e.g., "A baby sheep is a 'serwasid'. That's a made-up word. I know that a baby sheep is called a lamb".

Repeat with another sentence that the child will know, e.g., "A baby amap is called a puppy".

Repeat with other sentences until the child is confidently identifying the nonsense word (Step 1) and looking for meaning in the sentence (Step 2).

After each word meaning is detected, write down how the meaning was determined and create a list of actions the child can take to help him understand new words as part of completing Step 2.

Give the list a name, e.g., 'the rules for working out word meanings'. Step 1 will be 'find the word I don't know' and Step 2 will be 'how I work out the meaning'.

Repeat this activity in exactly the same way but this time create sentences that use real words that the child does not know.

Move on to using longer texts in the next activity.

SCIP Phase 2: LP 4

Resource

LP 4.2 Understanding verbal inferences

Activity 3 Resource: Working out word meaning from context

A baby sheep is a *serwash*. A baby *amap* is called a puppy.

The man wore his *frob* because it was raining.

Johnny was *labbing* down the street when he saw Isobel.

The dog was *litting* so loudly all the children ran away.

I put strawberry *cof* on my toast for breakfast.

Leaves fall off the trees in the *Skotteral*.

Elephants have a very long *froity*.

Today it is *erthups* outside so I'm going to wear my big warm coat.

At school I write my work with a blue *rif*. The teacher marks our work with *droob* one.

Mustafa is a chef. He cooks wonderful *gotty*! My favourite *gloobernast* is sausages. I like to eat them with mashed *fetkur*.

I can hop on one *apior* very well, so I am going to enter the hopping race on *Trabbnent* day. I hope that I will win the gold *zopner*.

I look at my *bedition* to see what time it is. It is time to get ready to go to school. We always ride our *frenapints* to school. Mum says it's OK as long as we wear our helmets.

Mum is trying to *dutop* her car in the carpark. Dad wears *heldies* when he drives so he can see the road signs better. When I can drive, I would like to drive a big red *thopper* so I can take lots of friends to the seaside.

SCIP Phase 2: LP 4

LP 4.2 Understanding verbal inferences

Activity 4: Understanding inferences in short stories

Purpose and target

To help the child develop skills in listening actively to stories and making inferences from spoken texts.

Materials

Short oral stories from 'Reading Comprehension Key Stage 1' stories, 'Scholastic Literacy Skills Comprehension ages 5–7', or similar.

Stories from *Understanding Inference* by Marilyn Toomey or similar.

Questions requiring an inference linked to each short story (maximum of 3 inferences per story).

LP 4.2 Activity 4 Resource.

Procedure

Explain the task as learning to listen to stories and work things out by thinking about the words we know. Make links to previous activity to prepare the child for the 'puzzle' question(s).

Explain the task as listening to some stories and answering a 'puzzle' question(s) first. Explain that a 'puzzle' question is one that you need to work out from clues in the story.

Model using a short story/sentence and an easy inference question.

Present the question(s) and read it aloud.

Leave the question(s) on the table and start reading the story/sentence.

At the end of the story, discuss the question and the answer.

Explain where in the text the clue to the answer was and repeat this bit of the text. Explain the inference and how that helped to answer the question.

Create a map of the text and the question with thinking bubbles to show the inferences.

Repeat with increasingly longer texts, modelling how to work out each answer.

Let the child join in as much as he can but always make the links from the text to the answer explicit.

Record a few examples in the child's workbook along with any symbols and key words that have proved helpful in working out the puzzle questions.

Repeat with a few stories and note any particular needs the child has in making inferences and teach as necessary to support this level of work.

SCIP Phase 2: LP 4

Resource

LP 4.2 Understanding verbal inferences

Activity 4 Resource: Understanding inferences in short stories

Hedgehog story

A hedgehog does not look like any other creature we have in the countryside. All the other mammals we see, such as rabbits, mice, or rats, are covered in fur. A hedgehog's back is covered with prickles. A hedgehog sleeps for most of the day under a pile of dry leaves. A hedgehog has up to seven hoglets. They are born blind and with soft prickles. They feed on milk from their mother when they are young. When they become adults they eat snails, slugs, worms, and beetles.

Inference questions

1. why wouldn't other animals try to eat hedgehogs?
2. are hedgehogs nocturnal?
3. what are baby hedgehogs called?
4. what do baby hedgehogs eat?

Fairground story

It was a Saturday morning in July. Katie and Natalie were going on a trip to the funfair.

"I'm going to go on all the fast rides", said Natalie. "I can't wait to go on those aeroplanes that go up and down and round and round", said Katie. Just then the coach arrived. "Hurry up and get on girls", said Brown Owl. "It will take at least an hour to get to the fair".

When they arrived at the fair everyone gave a big cheer. "Now don't lose your money", said Brown Owl. "Remember we will meet by the entrance at three o'clock". "I'm hungry", said Katie. "Let's go and get some candyfloss". They each bought a stick of candyfloss and ate it quickly. Katie soon found the aeroplane ride. "Let's go on these", she said. Natalie wasn't sure if she wanted to go on the aeroplane ride. It looked very high. "Come on", said Katie. Natalie didn't want to be left behind, so she went on the ride. "This is great!" shouted Katie as they went up and down and round and round. Natalie didn't say anything. She was thinking that she would be glad to be back on the ground. Natalie and Katie went on a few more rides.

Then Katie found a bench and sat down. "I don't want to go on any more rides", said Katie. "I think I ate too much candyfloss".

Inference questions

1. was the fair nearby?
2. did Katie enjoy the aeroplane ride?
3. how did Katie feel after going on the rides?

SCIP Phase 2: LP 4

LP 4.3 Understanding stories

Activity 1: Understanding story maps

Purpose and target

To help the child understand that stories can be broken down into different elements; and be able to answer questions on key factors such as characters, main events, purpose, motivations, and resolutions.

Materials

Short stories from 'Reading Comprehension Key Stage 1' stories or 'Scholastic Literacy Skills Comprehension ages 5–7' (or similar).

Child's own reading book and similar level texts from school.

Blank card to make a story map or Black Sheep Press Narrative Resources, or similar.

Procedure

Explain the task as learning to understand how stories fit together and to create a visual map to represent all the components of a story to make sure that you understand it.

Read a very short story within the child's needs and ability.

At the end, read each sentence separately and make a note of what story component was presented. Add a word or a symbol to the chart for this component, e.g., "James was in his bedroom". This sentence tells us *who is in the story and where he is.*

Work through the story sentence by sentence and map out the components together, drawing or writing out elements of the story as needed to ensure the child understands the task.

After you complete the story map, go back through the story and see if it makes sense and all events have been accounted for.

Read another few stories within the child's ability and each time allow the child to join in as much as he can but always make the links from the text to the map explicit.

Ensure that he can complete the story map with some independence before moving on to longer or more complex stories.

Include stories with inferences and work into the map a new step of how to map non-stated information, e.g., 'things I worked out'.

Record a few examples and a copy of the story map in the child's workbook.

Meta-challenge

When the child is confident, leave out a main event or detail and support him to notice that you 'forgot' this piece of information if he does not spot this independently.

SCIP Phase 2: LP 4

LP 4.3 Understanding stories

Activity 2: Predicting endings

Purpose and target

To develop the child's ability to integrate information from oral stories and make predictions for how the story can end.

Materials

Stories selected from 'Reading Comprehension Key Stage 1' stories, 'Scholastic Literacy Skills Comprehension ages 5-7' or *Telling a Story* by Marilyn M Toomey (or similar).

Story map created in LP 4.3 Activity 1.

Procedure

Explain the task as listening to stories and learning how to work out what might happen at the end.

Start with a simple story and stop before the end. Use the story map created in LP 4.3 Activity 1 to mark off the events that have been told, as before.

Review what is known about this story by talking through the story map.

Demonstrate how to work out the upcoming events by talking through and remembering all the things that have been told.

Discuss with the child the important events and what predictions can be made for each event.

Decide an ending and explain why this works for this story.

Meta-challenge

To emphasise the need for coherence, repeat using the same story but this time suggest an ending that does not fit, e.g., a new character appears, or any impossible or confusing ending.

Explain why this ending does not work and make a revised ending and compare.

Repeat with a few more stories, each time allowing the child to join in as much as he can but always make the links from the text to the predicted ending explicit.

Include stories with inferences and work into the ending an event that is derived from an inference.

Meta-challenge

When the child is becoming confident, repeat but suggest an impossible ending (meta-challenge) and ask him to explain why this won't work or support him to notice the mismatch if he does not spot this independently.

When using stories with inferences, make a false prediction by not including the inferred information and support the child as needed to detect and correct the mismatch.

SCIP Phase 2: LP 4

LP 4.3 Understanding stories

Activity 3: Looking back for information

Purpose and target

To help the child use the strategy of looking back at the picture or text of a story to check information and to engage actively in building representations of stories.

Materials

Create stories of suitable length and complexity, typed using double-spacing over up to three pages. Each page should have some text and a picture. Select suitable stories from resources such as the 'Reading Comprehension Key Stage 1' stories, 'Scholastic Literacy Skills', or similar

Comprehension ages 5–7 years or from school reading books at an age-appropriate level.

Questions associated with each story, some of which require inference.

Procedure

Explain the task as learning how to answer questions about stories and learning how to 'look back' at the story to get the answers. Explain that some answers will be remembered and some you will have to 'look back' in the story to find the answer.

Present the first story and read it aloud.

Ask a simple question that the child will probably be able to remember.

Explain that he knows the answer because "you can remember".

Ask another question that the child will probably not remember.

Explain that this usually happens: Some things are easy to remember and some things we need to 'check' by 'looking back'. Emphasise these words.

Support the child to hold the question in his head and show him how to look back at the text to find the answer. If necessary, write the question down and explain why this helps.

Re-read the paragraph that answers the question. Point out that the same words are in the question and the answer and that this can help find the answer in the text.

Work through the remaining questions about the story together, supporting the child as needed to look back at the story to find the answers.

Each time you ask the question, ask the child to state whether he can remember the answer or needs to 'look back' to emphasise and teach the name of the 'look back' strategy.

Repeat with a few more stories each time allowing the child to join in as much as he can but always make the steps to finding the answers explicit.

Meta-challenge

Suggest an incorrect answer and ask the child to explain why this is not correct and prove it by finding the right answer in the text.

Support as needed with strategies for working memory (LP 4.1 Activity 1) or comprehension monitoring (LP 5.1 Activity 1).

SCIP Phase 2: LP 4

LP 4.3 Understanding stories

Activity 4: Making mental maps of stories

Purpose and target

To help the child understand how to build mental representations of stories to assist comprehension and to develop awareness of how this helps comprehension.

Note: This is a challenging activity, but children aged eight years and above should be able to attempt it.

Materials

Resources as used in LP 4.3 Activity 3; create a composite picture for each story.

Procedure

Read a story aloud and at the end show the composite picture. Explain that 'making up a picture' about a story helps us to remember it and answer the questions. Emphasise these words.

Ask the questions and encourage the child to use the drawing to help.

Repeat with a new story and explain that this story doesn't have a picture and that he needs to make up a picture about the story in his mind.

If needed, start by visualising just one element of the story, e.g., the location or the people and gradually build up the complexity.

Read the start of the story aloud for the child and ask him to make a picture in his head for that person or event. Explain what needs to be included.

Add another piece of information and stop to make sure the child is adding to his mental picture of the story.

Ask the child some questions about the story and encourage him to use the picture in his mind to think about the answers.

Ask a simple question that the child will probably be able to answer.

Explain that he knows the answer because "you could make a picture in your head". Emphasise these words.

Ask another harder question and explain that it always happens like this: Some things are easy to remember and some things we need to go back and make a picture of the story in our heads.

Read the passage again and explain what the picture could look like.

If necessary, draw an image and explain why this helps.

Work through the questions about the story together, supporting the child as needed to make up images to support recall.

LP 1 Intervention content table

SCIP Phase 2	LP 5 Intervention content table

LP 5 Enhanced comprehension monitoring

LP 5 Information

LP 5.1 Text level comprehension monitoring

1 Comprehension monitoring and repairing in sentences plus Resource

LP 5.2 Task based comprehension monitoring

1 Asking for clarification in tasks

SCIP Phase 2: LP 5

Information

LP 5 Enhanced comprehension monitoring

The purpose of this Section is to help your child recognise when he has not understood any kind of spoken information, e.g., instructions, and to ask for clarification or repetition to support understanding.

This Section builds on work completed in Phase 1 when your child was taught to ask for repetition when instructions were deliberately delivered too quickly, too quietly, with a word missing, or when there was a competing noise. This helped your child understand that there are many reasons for not being able to follow spoken information and to build confidence in checking information rather than guessing. He has also practised asking for clarification when the instructions have been too long or have used words he doesn't know. A universal key phrase will have been taught, e.g., 'I don't know' or 'Tell me again'.

This Section builds on these core skills so that as tasks become more demanding your child can keep track of when he needs help and can ask more precisely for clarification, e.g., "Which child do you mean?", "Where shall I put the monkey?", "Tell me again. That was too long", "I don't know what that word means". The activities present increasingly complex instructions and support is provided to your child to engage confidently in self-help with regard to his/her understanding.

How you can help

Teaching in this Section will be tailored to meet your child's needs. Please be aware of and provide information on how your child currently reacts when he does not understand. All children experience times when they genuinely haven't understood in class or at home and will need support to ask for help at these times. Your child will need encouragement to use the positive strategies developed to assist in comprehension.

You can support your child to recognise when he hasn't understood by asking him explicitly after you have given some information, e.g., "Do you know what to do?" or "Shall I tell you again?".

Pictures and symbols for 'I know'/'I don't know' and 'asking for help' can be used at home and in class as a reminder. When you notice that your child has not understood but is not yet asking for clarification, you can explain what has happened, e.g., "I think that was 'too much information'" and be explicit when you repair it, saying, e.g., "I will tell you one thing at a time. That will make it easier for you".

Sometimes it will be possible to wait a few seconds longer than usual when you see he is confused. By using a clear facial expression or phrase to encourage him to ask for clarification ("If you need help, you can ask me"), your child can become more active. Use a light tone and lots of praise when your child does stop and ask.

SCIP Phase 2: LP 5

LP 5.1 Text level comprehension monitoring

Activity 1: Comprehension monitoring and repairing in sentences

Purpose and target

To assist the child to identify reasons for comprehension challenges in sentences and practise positive strategies for self-help.

Materials

Examples of sentences that contain an error in meaning from the Activity Resource 1. Highlighting pens and paper.

Procedure

Explain the task to the child as reading sentences and working out whether they make sense or have a mistake in them.

Explain that we need to read all the words to make sure that we understand what the sentence means.

Select one and read it aloud to the child.

Use the highlighting pens to highlight the two words whose meaning are in conflict.

Explain that both things cannot be true at the same time, e.g., old man and tenth birthday.

Re-write the sentence changing one of the words to make it make sense.

Highlight the two words that now make it sensible, e.g., old and ninety-first.

Change it again by changing old to young and man to boy and discuss as before.

Repeat and support the child to join in as you work through the list of sentences.

Include inferences in sentences, e.g., the man with grey hair and a walking stick instead of the old man to make the activity harder.

SCIP Phase 2: LP 5

Resource

LP 5.1 Text level comprehension monitoring

Activity 1 Resource: Comprehension monitoring and repairing in sentences

The old man celebrated his tenth birthday.

The boy opened the window to let his friend in.

The man parked his car in the living room.

Every night I look at the sun and count the stars.

My birthday is on the 42nd of May

I was late for school because my mum's television didn't go off this morning.

The teacher was so excited about her new school. She had a new school uniform and was really looking forward to playtime when she could meet some new friends.

My car keeps breaking down. I took it to the mechanic to get it fixed. He opened the bonnet and took the engine apart with a spoon.

John is a doctor, and he does operations on people's knees. He's a surgeon and he says, "I always put my paintbrushes away carefully at the end of the day".

Alex is a journalist. He packs his bag every morning after breakfast. This morning his wife spilt milk into his bag. She said, "Oh no, I'm sorry, I spilt milk on your stethoscope".

Valerie has toothache. She went to the dentist, and she recommended a new toothpaste called DOG FANG. It's for sensitive teeth.

David and his team of builders are building a new chapter on the side of my house. I can't wait for it to be finished. I'm going to sit in there and listen to music and look out all of the windows.

SCIP Phase 2: LP 5

LP 5.2 Task based comprehension monitoring

Activity 1: Asking for clarification in tasks

Purpose and target

To develop the child's ability to ask for clarification in tasks which require listening to instructions.

Materials

Construction game or making an object which involves listening to long or complicated instructions, e.g., simple origami tasks, building a robot.

All materials to make the object or play the game.

Prepare in advance a set of easy and complicated instructions for this task.

Requests for clarification written on to individual cards from Phase 1 CM.

Procedure

Hold back some of the craft materials or pieces of the game and use instructions that need these pieces early in the activity.

Begin the game and introduce it as one in which you will give instructions to make an object.

Say, "I'm going to give you some instructions that are easy to understand and some that are harder to understand".

Explain that the cards have good ways of asking for help written on them and that he can use these if he doesn't know what to do. Talk these through.

Get started by giving straightforward instructions.

Give an instruction that is either too long, confusing, or impossible because a piece of equipment is missing.

Explain why the instruction was too hard and use the matching request for clarification card.

Support the child to make a request for clarification using the written cards.

Repeat this activity using craft or games the child likes and explain that sometimes we need to ask for help when we are working on craft activities or playing games with friends.

Repeat with more complicated games and craft activities with more steps and unfamiliar vocabulary so that the child is monitoring comprehension in many ways in the same task.

INTERVENTION PLANNING AND RECORD FORM

Social Communication Intervention Programme

Catherine Adams and Jacqueline Gaile

SCIP	Assessment	**Personal information**	
Name: **Gender:**		**Date of birth/age:**	
Dates of assessment: **Dates of Intervention phases:**		**Speech-language practitioner:**	
School contact details: **Staff:**		**Preferred means of communication (parent):** Email/phone/Home-School Book	

SCIP	Assessment	**Individualised Social Communication Profile (ISCP)**

Section 1: List events in the child's typical day/week, interests, sports and activities, names of siblings, friends, pets, and important people. Give examples of events that are associated with specific emotions in the child (happy, sad, angry, scared).

Section 2: Summarise here information from parent discussion and teacher report, making reference to specific social situations the child finds challenging. Ask parents/teacher to provide a brief description of how the child reacts in the situation or interaction and ask them to describe changes they would like the child to be able to make for each situation.

DOI: 10.4324/9781032706641-7

379

SCIP	Assessment	**Assessment findings**
		Carry out assessment and observations and summarise below into the three main Components of SCIP Intervention. Record your impressions of overall strengths and needs in social communication, pragmatics, and language processing (receptive and expressive).

Social Understanding and Social Interpretation

Pragmatics

Language processing: Comprehension and expressive language and above-sentence-level skills

Other comments and observations, e.g., additional needs, behavioural observations

SCIP	Planner	**Priorities for intervention**

Ask parents/teachers to state their priorities for intervention in social communication.

SCIP Phase 1	Planner	**Planning delivery of Phase 1**

Add Phase 1 Objective codes for each block of intervention (3 sessions).

Block 1	**Block 2**

SCIP	Planner	**SCIP-GAS planning (Phase 2)**

Write agreed SCIP-GAS goals, scales used, and interim points on each scale here if used

SCIP Phase 1	Record	Progress in Phase 1 and indications for Phase 2
Record observations and progress from Phase 1 and make indications for Phase 2 plan and priorities.		
Phase 1 Objectives		**Progress and indications for Phase 2 planning**
Comprehension monitoring (CM)		
CM 1: Understanding the concept of knowing and not knowing		
CM 2: Understanding the concepts of guessing and working out		
CM 3: Strategies to signal non-comprehension		
CM 4: Asking for repetition		
Introduction to understanding social context (USC)		
USC 1: Making simple inferences from familiar sequences		
USC 2: Identifying social context from behaviours and language		
USC 3: Describing behaviours and language for social contexts		
USC 4: Simple personal reflection		
Basic metapragmatic awareness (MPA)		
MPA 1: Listening for content		
MPA 2: Understanding behaviours associated with listening		
MPA 3: Developing metapragmatic vocabulary		
MPA 4: Listener–speaker role-play		
Basic narrative (BN)		
BN 1: Understanding vocabulary for sequencing		
BN 2: Making simple inferences from pictures		
BN 3: Simple sequencing		
BN 4: Simple personal stories		
Introduction to emotions in context (EM)		
EM 1: Matching pictures and symbols to facial expressions		
EM 2: Linking emotions to events		
EM 3: Emotions ladder		
EM 4: Making inferences from facial expression and eye gaze		

SCIP Phase 2	Planner	**Social Understanding and Social Interpretation (SUSI)**
Use the Assessment to Intervention Map to select SUSI Sections to be included in Phase 2. Record findings against each Section. Use prioritisation guidelines and observations and progress in Phase 1 to indicate starting points and priorities.		

SUSI Intervention content	Assessment findings and observations from Phase 1
SUSI 1 Understanding social context cues in interactions	
SUSI 1.1 Understanding non-verbal cues in context	
SUSI 1.2 Understanding and solving problems in simple contexts	
SUSI 2 Understanding emotion cues in interactions	
SUSI 2.1 Building emotion vocabulary	
SUSI 2.2 Enhanced emotion vocabulary	
SUSI 2.3 Understanding complex feelings	
SUSI 3 Understanding and practising flexibility	
SUSI 3.1 Understanding routines	
SUSI 3.2 Understanding and coping with unplanned change	
SUSI 3.3 Making changes in personal routines	
SUSI 4 Understanding thoughts and intentions of others	
SUSI 4.1 Signalling feelings and intentions (non-verbal)	
SUSI 4.2 Predicting thoughts and intentions	
SUSI 4.3 Understanding mismatch of language and thoughts	
SUSI 4.4 Understanding complex intentions	
SUSI 5 Understanding friendship	
SUSI 5.1 Understanding interests in friendship	
SUSI 5.2 Understanding the impact of preferred interests	
SUSI 5.3 Understanding friendship skills	

SCIP Phase 2	Planner	**Pragmatics (PRAG)**

Use the Assessment to Intervention Map to select PRAG Sections to be included in Phase 2. Record findings against each Section. Use prioritisation guidelines and observations and progress in Phase 1 to indicate starting points and priorities.

PRAG Intervention content	Assessment findings and observations from Phase 1
PRAG 1 Turn-taking and reciprocity	
PRAG 1.1 Understanding how to take turns	
PRAG 1.2 Understanding verbal turn-taking	
PRAG 1.3 Consolidating turn-taking skills	
PRAG 2 Conversation and metapragmatic skills	
PRAG 2.1 Enhanced listening skills	
PRAG 2.2 Understanding speaker roles	
PRAG 2.3 Giving information	
PRAG 2.4 Developing metapragmatic awareness	
PRAG 3 Understanding information requirements	
PRAG 3.1 Understanding impact of missing information	
PRAG 3.2 Understanding impact of too much information	
PRAG 3.3 Understanding matching context and talk	
PRAG 3.4 Understanding information requirements in personal conversation	
PRAG 4 Understanding and managing topic in conversation	
PRAG 4.1 Identifying topics	
PRAG 4.2 Understanding topic change conventions	
PRAG 4.3 Consolidating topic skills	
PRAG 5 Understanding and improving discourse style	
PRAG 5.1 Understanding different styles in interaction	
PRAG 5.2 Understanding and using conventions of interaction style	
PRAG 5.3 Consolidating interaction style	

SCIP Phase 2	Planner	Language Processing (LP)	

Use the Assessment to Intervention Map to select LP Sections to be included in Phase 2. Record findings against each Section. Use prioritisation guidelines and observations and progress in Phase 1 to indicate starting points and priorities.

LP Intervention content	Assessment findings and observations from Phase 1
LP 1 Vocabulary and word knowledge	
LP 1.1 Understanding semantic relationships between words	
LP 1.2 Consolidation and self-cueing	
LP 1.3 Vocabulary enrichment	
LP 2 Narrative construction	
LP 2.1 Understanding inferences in picture sequences	
LP 2.2 Telling complex and personalised stories	
LP 2.3 Constructing novel stories with plots	
LP 3 Non-literal language	
LP 3.1 Understanding homophones	
LP 3.2 Understanding literal and non-literal meanings	
LP 3.3 Understanding non-literal meanings in context	
LP 4 Discourse comprehension	
LP 4.1 Improving memory and listening	
LP 4.2 Understanding verbal inferences	
LP 4.3 Understanding stories	
LP 5 Enhanced comprehension monitoring	
LP 5.1 Text level comprehension monitoring	
LP 5.2 Task based comprehension monitoring	

SCIP Phase 2	Planner	Block planner and goals
Add the goals for Phase 2. Add the Section or Objective codes for each session.		
Phase 2 goals		

Session 1	Session 2	Session 3
Session 4	Session 5	Session 6
Session 7	Session 8	Session 9
Session 10	Session 11	Session 12
Session 13	Session 14	Session 15
Session 16	Session 17	Session 18

SCIP Phase 3	Planner	**Phase 3 Personalised goals**

Using information from the ISCP and with reference to progress in Phase 2 Sections, select up to three situations to be supported to generalise in Phase 3. Record the child's current interaction and develop a personalised goal based on progress in Phase 2 and parent/teacher preferences for change. List the Phase 2 Objectives relevant to the success of each goal and ensure these have been mastered.

Social communication situation 1

Describe the situation	
Child's current interaction	
Personalised goal for this situation	
Phase 2 Objectives relevant to this goal	

Social communication situation 2

Describe the situation	
Child's current interaction	
Personalised goal for this situation	
Phase 2 Objectives relevant to this goal	

Social communication situation 3

Describe the situation	
Child's current interaction	
Personalised goal for this situation	
Phase 2 Objectives relevant to this goal	

SCIP Phase 3	Planner	**Phase 3 Personalised activity**

Write the Phase 3 goal, materials, and procedure detailing how meta-challenges and naturally occurring mismatches will be discussed in the priming and personalised stages of the activity.

Activity title

Phase 3 goal

Materials

Procedure (Context for priming activity and meta-challenge response)

Procedure (Context for personalised activity and response to naturally occurring mismatches)

Success criteria

SCIP Phase 2	Assessment to Intervention Map	Short version
Identify which Sections of Phase 2 Intervention should be included in the Planner		

Guidance for inclusion	Phase 2 Sections
Can misinterpret social situations, makes mismatched comments, may misunderstand social cues within context	SUSI 1 Understanding social context cues in interactions
Has needs in understanding and expressing emotions in context, may not recognise non-verbal cues	SUSI 2 Understanding emotion cues in interactions
Prefers routine and sameness, change needs to be carefully managed, unplanned change is upsetting	SUSI 3 Understanding and practising flexibility
Challenges in making verbal or social inferences, does not understand deception, tricks, or jokes, unintentionally hurtful	SUSI 4 Understanding thoughts and intentions of others
Finds it hard to join in with his peer group, isolated in playground	SUSI 5 Understanding friendship
Does not relinquish or take up turns in conversation, needs in reciprocity, and turn-taking. Can be difficult to interrupt talk	PRAG 1 Turn-taking and reciprocity
Conversational flow shows some misunderstandings which the child cannot clarify. May not initiate or ask questions, may not recognise non-verbal signals to start or stop talking	PRAG 2 Conversation and metapragmatic skills
Includes very precise information, but also talks about things either not established or already known. Referents are sometimes unclear	PRAG 3 Understanding information requirements
Preferred topics dominate conversation, unaware of others' level of interest, does not signal topic change, lists facts	PRAG 4 Understanding and managing topic in conversation
Changing style to match different types of interactions is challenging, can appear overly formal or familiar in conversation	PRAG 5 Understanding and improving discourse style
Naming subtest score/performance indicative of word finding needs, evidence of neologisms, or mismatches in word choices in narrative or conversation	LP 1 Vocabulary and word knowledge
Narrative test scores outside the expected range with needs in recounting events in order or in detail	LP 2 Narrative construction
Understanding of similes, metaphors, homophones, and idioms shows characteristics associated with younger children	LP 3 Non-literal language
Inferential comprehension needs; shows needs in comprehension of complex sentences, text or conversation from formal testing or report of performance at home/school	LP 4 Discourse comprehension
Practitioner observations from Phase 1 Comprehension monitoring indicates need for further work	LP 5 Enhanced comprehension monitoring

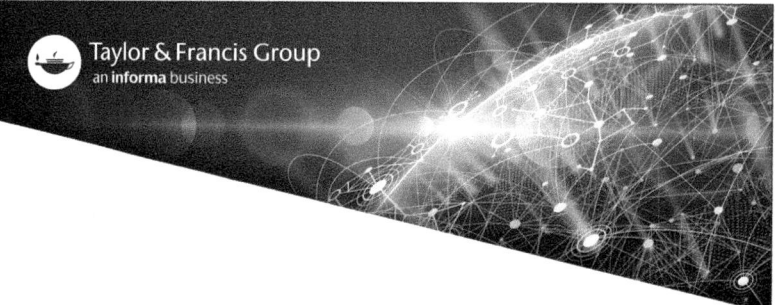
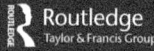
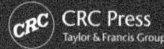